THE HEALING ADVENTURE

As a practicing physician, I have been acquainted with the Cayce material and working with it at the clinical level since 1957. As Director of the Edgar Cayce Foundation Medical Research Division, it has been my privilege to study the concepts of body function described in these readings, to see results come about from application of principles found there, and to correspond with many A.R.E. (Association for Research and Enlightenment) members concerning questions of their health and manners in which they themselves have been using the material they found in the readings. . . .

The physical is our present state of existence, and Cayce directed most of his suggestions about healing toward the physical body. And he seemed to be saying that the process we go through in being healed of our physical and mental disabilities is an adventure in consciousness.

So, on with the adventure!

—William A. McGarey, M.D.

CONTENTS

This book is dedicated to Hugh Lynn Cayce, who died July 4, 1982. More than any other person, Hugh Lynn was responsible for the growth of the Cayce work; and it was Hugh Lynn who stimulated me to work with these concepts of healing which have made this book possible.

ACKNOWLEDGMENTS

The making of this book dates back twenty-five years, to what I call the early days on the road, lecturing on health, dreams, home, and marriage, and the various Edgar Cayce phenomena. Elsie and Bill Sechrist urged me to call it "What to Do Until the Spontaneous Remission Comes," for they had been with Gladys and me through many trips, many talks, and many experiences.

But it was really through my experiences with the concepts in the Edgar Cayce readings on health and healing that the book came into being. Hugh Lynn Cayce urged me over and over again to work on the physical readings his dad gave. And he counseled me in writing and in living up to the advice I would give in writing. Gladys Davis Turner has always been a source of inspiration, help, and information during and since the summer of 1967, when I was working at Virginia Beach writing some twenty-five medical commentaries.

The doctors I've worked with, the thousands of patients with whom I have sought to solidify the concepts of healing we were working with, the many secretaries who have worked with me over the years, the staff at the A.R.E. Clinic—all of these have been my teachers. But there has always been that incessant drive inside myself to write, and I had to write something that was meaningful—something that would change other people's lives. I found this in the Cayce readings, and that was undoubtedly the most important factor in my writing this book.

I could not have written it without my wife Gladys's constant encouragement, faith, steadfastness, and her telling me that my writing was excellent, even though I knew in my heart it often was not. It takes editing to make the best of most writing efforts, and Richard I. Abrams, with his fine mind and sensitive spirit, provided that final touch.

There are unknown hundreds of correspondents who have contributed to my experiences and to this book. I can't name them, but I thank them, as I would thank everyone who might find life better as a result of reading these pages.

PREFACE

I first met Dr. William McGarey in 1965 in Virginia Beach, Virginia, at the headquarters of the Association for Research and Enlightenment (A.R.E.), which houses the voluminous files containing the transcripts of the Edgar Cayce psychic readings.

Bill McGarey told how, in 1955, ten years after Cayce's death, he began to take an interest in Cayce's health readings. Making his own diagnoses, he began treating difficult cases with castor oil packs and other Cayce remedies. Amazingly, they worked.

Some fifteen years after that, McGarey launched a clinic in Phoenix, Arizona, specializing in Cayce-type treatments. Since then, more than thirty thousand patients of all types and ages have passed through his clinic.

I have known several of these patients. All received treatments like those recommended years before by Cayce for similar ailments. In each case the patient got better. One, a small boy, was cured of a bronchial asthmatic condition that defied conventional therapy and threatened his life. Another, an elderly woman, was treated for "incurable" cancer as Cayce would have proposed, with equal attention to body, mind, and spirit. Now, ten years later, the woman is more hale and hearty than ever.

Originally, there were only McGarey and his wife, Gladys, who is also a medical doctor, and a handful of aides. Now there are nearly forty people, including physicians, primary care staff, nurses, therapists, technicians, researchers, and backup personnel. The present facility is itself a holistic Center for Wellness, with biofeedback, music therapy, and educational and research programs in nutrition, exercise, meditation, and the nature of illness itself. A spacious Center for Regeneration is planned in a beautiful desert terrain in Casa Grande, forty miles from Phoenix.

Long before McGarey came on the scene, Dr. Wesley Ketcham worked directly with Cayce to help people whom ordinary therapy didn't help. Their relationship lasted several years. When it ended, a marveling Ketcham advised Cayce: "A hundred years from now doctors will be reading what you said and treating patients as you prescribed." Let it be known that Dr. McGarey was one of those who made a prophet of Ketcham.

Malibu, California   Jess Stearn
January 1983

INTRODUCTION

It was more than seventy-five years ago that Edgar Cayce gave his first reading—a discourse about his own health from a state of mind and body that some have called a trance, some an extended state of consciousness. Cayce died in 1945, leaving for study a body of information that emanated from his unconscious mind and that covered subjects ranging from prehistory to predicted earth changes.

Most of his work, however, had to do with the human body and its illnesses, its nature and its healing capabilities. Out of the 14,879 readings that are recorded and indexed in the library of the Association for Research and Enlightenment in Virginia Beach, Virginia, 8,968 were given for individuals who were concerned about their physical welfare.

As a practicing physician, I have been working with the Cayce material at the clinical level since 1957. As Director of the Edgar Cayce Foundation Medical Research Division, it has been my privilege to study the concepts of body function described in these readings, to see results come about from application of principles found there, and to correspond with many A.R.E. members concerning questions of their health and manners in which they themselves have been using the material they found in the readings.

The approach to health and healing found in the Cayce material is best termed *holistic*—for, over and over again, in his sleeping state, Cayce saw the human being as a whole entity in time and space. "The spirit is the life, the mind is the builder, and the physical is the result." This seems to be the theme of Cayce's assessment of man's state here on Earth. He saw man as a traveler in time and space, a stranger on Earth, having his origin and his destiny in a spiritual realm, which we perceive most often only through the inner eyes and the words of those who have been given that privilege. So it is that each of us is an eternal being, having existed in a form that is self-conscious prior to birth, and continuing that existence when the physical body dies.

Yet, the physical is our present state of existence, and Cayce directed most of his suggestions about healing toward the physical body. He seemed to be saying that the process we go through in being healed of our physical and mental disabilities is an adventure in consciousness.

So, on with the adventure!

This book will not be an exhaustive study of Cayce's work—the material in the readings is much too diverse and expansive to do that. Instead, I will discuss ideas that have become part of my way of life in the practice of medicine, and will describe how healing comes about, as I see it. I will also explore creative discoveries of others who, not being physicians, have put into action concepts of healing or simple modalities of therapy that Cayce described at one time or another.

Part One is a section on ideas, concepts, and the nature of man and healing. Part Two describes procedures and ideas for healing the body. Part Three focuses on specific areas of the body where ill health resides. Finally, Part Four, the conclusion, sums up the material presented, bringing it more into a whole.

Finally, my success and that of others with the healing techniques described here may not apply to every reader. Treatments should be taken or administered after consultation with or supervision by a doctor or other trained person.

It would be proper to say that this book is about healing; and healing, in the final analysis, is everybody's business: from the mother who kisses her little boy's hurt finger and makes it better, to the surgeon who removes a life-threatening "hot" appendix. We all take part in healing the human body.

Part One
THE SETTING

Chapter One
WHAT IS THE HUMAN BODY?
WHY ILLNESS?

When I was an eight-year-old boy, I frequently looked up into the night sky, saw all those wonderful sparkling stars, and wondered how far out space really went. I knew from school that distances out there were measured in lightyears, not miles, and that the farthest star that had been studied must be billions of lightyears distant from our planet Earth. But how far was that? And, when you got to the end of space, what was beyond that?

It boggled my mind—and, in my more mature years, I have come to the conclusion that space must not be a three-dimensional unit. It must be something like the source of all things we call God—simply not understandable by our present, limited mental functioning.

The human body and its mystery is like space and its infinitude, like the atom and its vastness, for we understand none of these with our present, finite minds—even as we understand God only partially and our own spiritual nature with dimness of vision. But it is our challenge to charge ahead and try to understand as we go about our daily tasks in life— and my tasks have moved me toward that mystery we call the human body, with its illnesses and its need to be healed and made whole.

In his extended state of consciousness, Edgar Cayce saw illness and health related to right action and error; but it was all superimposed on a cosmic plan that placed man in the center of things, with a spiritual origin and a spiritual destiny. From Cayce's source of information, and from the Old Testament story, man was created as a spiritual being before this universe came into existence.

Rabbi Herbert Weiner, an authority on the Kabala,

the Jewish book of wisdom, likes to tell the Kabala story about the Angel of Forgetfulness. It seems that everyone, prior to his birth, is given a chance to see what is going to happen to him. The Angel of Forgetfulness takes the individual to a special place and shows him all the important future events in his life if he chooses to be born at that time. If he chooses to go ahead, the Angel then touches him on the center of the upper lip, he forgets everything that he saw, and he is born.

Whether or not events are exactly like that (and you will have to decide—unless you remember), it is without doubt a beneficial thing that we cannot foresee the future. We have enough difficulty keeping up with the present without seeing what is in store for us—even though at that time we might have accumulated a bit more experience and hopefully a lot more wisdom.

Looking into the past is another matter. Assuming that we have lived many lifetimes to contribute to our present state of being, the past, as we understand it, is already finished and can be met again only in reaping the harvest of what we have done or sown. This law is called karma, or the law of cause and effect. However, the past is gone.

So, it is part curiosity and part for purposes of understanding and learning that many seek information about past lives and what happened in the dim, dark regions of ages long ago. The *life readings*, which provide a significant portion of the Cayce material, give much helpful information about past lives. Today—unlike times even in the recent past—people are remembering more and more past life experiences, and there are many individuals who can give the seeker a past life reading.

In the field of healing, one cannot bring about a true change unless he takes into account the ongoing experience of life that one moves through over the period of many incarnations . . . that is, if reincarnation really happens. I have taken the position that it does.

Illness and health often have their inception in past lives. Tendencies of the emotions arise in the glands that are the repositories of memories of past lives. Such tendencies lead unerringly toward a lack of balance, or a greater degree of balance, which spells either disease or better health. Understanding these tendencies, putting up with the karmic physical hangovers, helps us to be patient with ourselves as we seek better health and a reawakened consciousness.

We can then say that we are spiritual beings, gifted with minds and bodies, who have experienced past lives here on Earth, and who are part of an ongoing living process, seeking the direction that will lead us toward that goal that instinctively we know is our spiritual destiny.

A pathological condition does not appear miraculously or all at once. It develops in a process that takes time. Some conditions tell a story about their beginnings and their development, and without these bits of reality somewhere in the body, a disease could not come into existence. Disease does not exist outside the body. Pathogens, bacteria, viruses, and carcinogens do have reality when not in contact with the body, but the diseases they cause are only potential, and the so-called disease-producing factors never create disease one hundred percent of the time. Within the body are all the natural defenses, which in most cases protect the body against disease organisms.

Probably the most important point to be aware of in the prevention of disease is that these protective mechanisms inherent within each human body can be deficient, but they can be strengthened. The critical moments come about when, due to disturbing activity of the mind or the emotions, or perhaps through lack of care about the needs of the body itself (such as diet, exercise, and sleep), there is a suppression of the defenses, and the door is opened, so to speak, to the disease process.

Once a beginning is made, there is a progression of the disease toward serious and sometimes life-threatening illness. However, the disease may be interrupted or reversed at any point, and the return to normal functioning may be rapid, or it may occur over a long period of time. Sometimes, the return or healing may be almost instantaneous. Nevertheless, the nature of disease is fundamentally a process, because man—also a progression in the span of time—is where disease takes place.

The idea that man is body, mind, and spirit, and that all three are one, in a very real sense, needs to be recognized and dealt with each time the patient comes into contact with the physician, the healer, the therapist, the nurse, or the front-office personnel. When one is looking for the cause of the disease and searching for the best therapy program, this holistic concept of the human being needs recognition and appreciation.

Within the concepts of the Edgar Cayce readings, it is often repeated that illness is sin, or being out of harmony and not experiencing at-oneness with God. If all illness is sin, then we must ask just what Cayce meant when he worked with that activity in the lives of men. According to Cayce, a person may need castor oil—if he is in a castor oil consciousness; or he may benefit most from penicillin—if he is in a penicillin consciousness. A diathermy treatment may be his choice in order to come to a healing, or surgery may be necessary—all due to the nature of his consciousness. It is no wonder that there are so many ways to arrive at the state we call healing. Further, if we can use physical means to overcome sickness, which is sin, then we should also be able to use mental means and spiritual aids in reversing the pathological process.

As we look at man's experience over many lifetimes, and the illnesses that are built out of the law of cause and effect, is it possible to reverse these processes through fruits of the spirit or through physical aids? This is a question that everyone who is acquainted with the idea of reincarnation must ask. Through my research of the Cayce readings, I have come to the conclusion that most of the serious, long-term, degenerative diseases are karmic in their nature: Parkinson's disease, rheumatoid arthritis, amyotrophic lateral sclerosis, muscular dystrophy, and the like. There are seemingly contradictory points of view expressed in the world literature, the Bible, and in the Cayce readings as to the potential reversibility of such diseases.

To the physician it is essential that conclusions to the question of reversibility be drawn, for they would have a strong bearing on how a patient is to be treated. For example, if one carries to a logical conclusion the statement in the Bible that "He who kills with the sword will die by the sword" (Rev. 13:10), then the karma that afflicts the body must fulfill its course. There are many other citable instances that would lead one to assume that it would be fruitless to seek a full return to normal in a real karmic condition.

However, there is always a point where karma ceases and, like any "debt," is paid off. There is no law that the debt must be paid off only when a person dies in the physical body, carrying his disease process with him to the end. There is always a point where karma ends, and it seems that this is the point where spiritual understanding occurs, or where the "lesson" is learned. This juncture might be called "Where Karma Ends and Grace Begins." For what we are calling grace seems to be that point at which forgiveness is accepted *by the person experiencing the karma.* Such self-forgiveness may have been offered for a long time, but the self-acceptance may have been rejected. The Cayce readings appear to lend credence to the concept that such rejection is rebellion, and rebellion is sin, as is the disease. Thus, the self-acceptance must be a portion of the healing process, and must be a part of the spiritual learning that an individual undergoes during his time on Earth.

If karmic forces can, then, be met in definite spiritual purposes, the physician working with "incurable" diseases is challenged to treat such patients as individuals who may at any moment have learned the lesson that brought about the illness experience. Accordingly, his treatment program must have a spiritual direction, and the mind must be engaged in bringing about the necessary educational process. The physician must work patiently with the patient who is trying to overcome what has become part of his total life experience.

As a physician, it becomes truly fascinating when one approaches the healing of the human body from the point of view of it being an adventure in an individual's total consciousness, and an opportunity to witness grace as it becomes active in the disease process.

Chapter Two

A CLOSER LOOK AT THE HUMAN BODY

We should inquire about this mystery that we call the human body. In the field of medicine, it becomes the central focus of research, although today it is probably not recognized as such. Indeed, in medicine today the pervasive emphasis is on the disease, studying the disease, measuring the disease, as if in reality the disease exists apart from the mystery and intricacies of the individual human being.

Medicine exists for the individual patient, and the greatest source of information is still to be found in that individual . . . and that patient is you and that patient is I. An editorial published some years ago in the *Journal of the Medical Society of New Jersey* (February 1973) 70:94, perhaps best sums up this point of view:

> The patient is really the fountainhead of all research. Imaginative people are always trying to dream up research projects. But they often leave untilled the one never-ending source of ideas and fountain of factual datum—the one we must know how to read. The patient is a book waiting to be read by a sensitive eye and an inspired mind. Every patient offers an opportunity for a fresh look at the facts. In the equations of medical research, he represents the unknowns, and con-

verting the unknown into the known is the goal
of medical research. If one appears to be worn out
by reviewing the same research questions, there
is strength to be found in going back to the prime
source: the patient.

In taking a closer look at the human body, it is
necessary to develop an understanding of what is
going on in the nervous system. Cayce saw the importance of electricity and its role in the functioning
of the human being. He described in many readings
the manner in which the nerve cells reach out, searching for new connections. He also delved further into
causation and discussed the source or nature of
electricity as it is found both inside and outside the
body:

> . . . for all Force, all power, *emanates* from one
> source. So, as has been given, that which makes
> up even the electronic energy—that man knows
> as electrons or energy in electricity, which may be
> used as a convenience, as a necessity for man's
> experience—is of God itself.
>
> 4757–1

In the readings, Cayce talks about the relationship
between the autonomic and the cerebrospinal nervous systems. He indicated that the autonomic nervous system mediated the unconscious mind and its
activities, while the cerebrospinal system was concerned with the conscious mind.

A key to understanding the body and its functions,
then, lies in knowing that electrical and electronic
impulses are basic to that functioning: primary in
thought, in sensing the world around us, in digestion and all the body activities, and in creating either constructive or destructive activities within our
lives. All these impulses must be coordinated within
the body or confusion and disruption occurs.

The concept of incoordination appears regularly
in the Edgar Cayce readings as he discusses physiological functioning in the human body. For me, this
idea has become a cornerstone in understanding

illness and health, for health simply cannot be obtained when organs or systems are not working together within the body. It is coordinant function that allows proper assimilation of foods and proper elimination of waste materials. When the nervous systems move out of phase with one another or become even slightly incoordinated, trouble arises, sometimes serious, sometimes minor in nature, but always trouble.

Cayce gave a great deal of understanding to the concept that there are three nervous systems in our bodies. This differs radically from what we are taught in medical school. Much is taught about the five senses and their importance, but in our books on physiology and anatomy they are not grouped together as a system that works as a unit, similar to the autonomic nervous system or the cerebrospinal nervous system. However, the Cayce readings do spell out just such an understanding, and it does make sense. Cayce suggested, for instance, that colors, perceived by the eye, have a greater impact on the autonomic nervous system and probably reach that area more quickly and definitely than they reach the cerebrospinal system—that is, the brain. We know today that colors do influence our emotions even when we are not consciously aware of them.

Not only in the nervous system itself does the body produce various states of incoordination, but it may come about between the functions of the organs. The eliminatory organs, for example, must work together or there is difficulty. The liver and gut, the skin, the lungs, and the kidneys all take care of a portion of the substances that must be eliminated from the body. If the kidneys fail, we call it uremia, a condition wherein those body residues that are normally eliminated by the kidneys are not able to be removed by any of the other organs of elimination. Continued far enough, such a buildup of body toxins spells death. Modern technology has made kidney dialysis and kidney transplants possible, but it has not yet solved the question as to why the kidney fails in the first place.

Much could be written on any of these subjects

dealing with the body and its functions, but it should
be noted that all organs of the body function not
only independently but in coordination with other
organs and with the body pattern taken as a whole.
It has always seemed to me that the body was designed in the first place to satisfy the needs of the
spiritual being we call man to live cooperatively with
and in this third dimension so that purposes could
be fulfilled. This means that all parts of the body
must work together for the good of the whole, and
no part can function totally independent of the rest.

Coordination might also be called balance. In the
human body the result of balance is homeostasis,
the condition of the body in which the living process
is allowed to continue without noticeable difficulty.

One of the manners in which the body assumes a
balance is in the acid-base, or acid-alkaline, relationship. I am more and more convinced that this kind
of balance, as it is expressed in the body tissues, is a
critical thing. We know that numerous tissues, fluids,
and tracts of the body depend upon their pH, or
acidity level, for normal function. The blood, for
example, must maintain a pH within a very limited
critical range or the body becomes seriously ill. The
vaginal tract, the lymph fluid, and the stomach
contents, to mention a few, must keep themselves at
specific levels of acidity or alkalinity to function properly and resist the inroads of disease.

If you eat something that is alkaline in its reaction
to the body, it will produce alkalinity that must be
eliminated from the body, or make the tissues more
alkaline, since the bloodstream remains remarkably
stable in this regard. Thus, excess acidity in the
diet, or caused by the way one thinks and emotes,
may produce acidity in tissues that may be weak or
under stress, rather than simply being eliminated
through the bladder or through the intestines.

If the stomach and small intestines perform their
proper function—assuming, of course, that the diet
is adequate—in digesting and assimilating necessary food substance; and if the eliminations of the
body are kept normal, so as to prevent any buildup
in toxic substances; and if the thoughts and emotions,

the environment and heredity, and the karmic influences are all constructive; then, it seems reasonable
to assume that the body-mind-spirit unity that we
call the human being will be healthy, at that given
moment in time.

However, this may not necessarily be the case. The
immune system may have suffered a blow at an
earlier time and not yet have recovered. This immune system is the thymus system and includes all
the lymphatic tissue in the body, the liver and spleen,
the thymus itself, the tonsils, the appendix, the
Peyer's patches,* and all the lymph nodes and lymphatic channels. This system is the subject of much
study in the areas of immunology and organ transplants. This system provides defenses for the entire
body and also is the primary eliminatory channel for
all the cells in the body. The lymph is always in
alkaline balance when it is in the state of health.

Cayce saw the lymphatics as being important in
taking from the ingested food certain values and
preparing them so that they "may be used to revivify,
revitalize, recharge the system itself." (1055–1) He
also saw other functions that he described and al-
luded to in his own terminology. Today these functions are described in terms of immunology—the
study of the protective influences of the body that
keep infections under control and thus prolong life.

When we consider that the entire body, with its
billions of cells (and how many atoms?), comes
into being from the union of two cells, the sperm
and the ovum, we can understand that we have in
the body an everchanging, magnificent creation that
defies a complete knowledge of it. The body is in one
sense a unity, for it speaks as one person. But it
also has many diverse activities and comes to be
either male or female.

Speaking of unit and polarity, Edgar Cayce once
stated that the process of creation, in a sense, is the
movement of substance in the spiritual coming into

---

*Peyer's patches are oval patches of lymphoid tissue found
in the walls of the small intestine, the duodenum, the
jejunum, and the ilium.

materiality by taking on polarity—negativity and positivity. The atom in the spiritual realm is a unity, but in the material world it has its positive and negative charges. Cayce also saw the atom as having consciousness, and in the middle of a physical reading he gave this information:

> . . . as we see, every atom of the body is as a whole universe or an element in itself. It either coordinates or it makes for disruptive forces by its activity being expelled from the system through the activity of the eliminating system. . . .
>
> 759—9

We are indeed remarkable creations, if these concepts are valid, and the sum total consciousness of one individual is a world unto itself.

Cayce was once asked, during the course of a reading, how one could develop the power to heal. He replied:

> . . . through Him who gives all force, all power as manifestations to individuals, that his glory may be manifest among men. As to the development of the power that is given, this depends upon whose glorification is being made manifest. Hence, one may possess much knowledge, much power, to one's own undoing. In using same, if self, self's desire, self's aims are made one with Him, *through* Him may much understanding come.
>
> 255—11

So, the inner wisdom of the body may be tapped, but there are requirements that must be met, if the course is to be taken in the right direction.

My wife, Dr. Gladys McGarey, for years has tapped this inner wisdom in her relationships with patients. For her, that knowledge lies inherent within the individual and shows up as the dream capacity. "I would like a consultation," the patient is told, "not with one of our local doctors, but with the physician within you!" There is the ability to draw from this inner knowledge in such a way that the instructions needed to diagnose or treat an illness may be brought to the surface—most commonly in a dream. A gentleman who was bothered with aches and pains in his joints told me this dream:

> I heard a knock at the door, and it was a kindly-looking old man who nodded to me, entered the house without being really invited, and motioned to me to follow him. He took me downstairs to the cellar, showed me the drainpipes to the bathrooms in the house, and told me that they were all plugged up and would hardly let the water through. That was the end of the dream.

It did not take the knowledge of a genius to interpret the dream as a sign that the eliminations of the body were in poor shape, and that they should be corrected, if the man would have a healthy body once more.

The communication from the unconscious realm to the conscious awareness comes most often in more complicated symbols, but the messages are always there for those who will look at the dream content and try to understand.

So it is by searching, by seeking to find the answer, whether it lies within our own consciousness or elsewhere, that we begin to gain an understanding of the body and its wonders, and the wisdom to seek healing in patience, persistence, and consistency.

Chapter Three
HEALING AND HEALTH

Ever since I started my practice of medicine more than thirty years ago, I have been fascinated by what we call the healing process. For, as we have already discovered, the human being is himself a living process, and a return to health must also be classified as a process.

In my searching, I have found that there are literally a multitude of methods championed as "the
ultimate" in bringing healing to the human body. In
my field of allopathic medicine, drugs, surgery, or
X-rays are used to lay low that process we call disease.
We pay precious little attention, really, to building
up the health of the body. Nutritionists, on the other
hand, act as if the right combination of foods and
vitamins will cure anything. Hynotists bring about
reversals of body conditions almost miraculously at
times. Acupuncturists, osteopaths, and chiropractors all feel that their method of healing is the ultimate answer.

Those who have attended a Kathryn Kuhlman service or made a pilgrimage to the French shrine at
Lourdes may have let go of all other therapies, expecting these to be the final cure. I could go on—
herbs, Christian Science, Unity, homeopathy, physical
therapy, laying on of hands, prayer therapy. There
are, indeed, many ways to bring about a better condition of health in the body.

As a physician, I have been interested in how a
state of harmony often comes about in the patient
as he seeks professional help. Harmony is consistent with health, and health is exactly what the
patient is seeking.

It is not just the physician, of course, who offers
this kind of therapy. I have had patients tell me, "I
don't know why it is, but as soon as I come into the
Clinic, I feel better." Is it the smile of the receptionist?
Is it the warmth of the nurse? Is it the confidence
that is inspired by the people involved? Whatever
this elusive magic is that we loosely call healing, it
has to do with the Spirit of Life itself, as it is manifested in the people who are seeking help and in
those who are offering it.

In the Cayce material concerning the healing
process, the matter of consciousness keeps coming
up. This has always seemed reasonable to me, for
our entire adventure through a lifetime here on Earth
is an adventure in consciousness. Healing of the
body should certainly be a similar adventure. Cayce
pointed out that even an atom can be made aware of

the influence that would regenerate or rebuild the body itself. Perhaps it is when this awareness really comes about that healing occurs.

Healing of the body is always to some extent a regeneration of tissue, although it is generally understood in the field of medicine that the only true regeneration within the human body comes about in the healing of bone after a fracture. The fractured bone is brought into alignment as closely as possible; then the body goes through the procedure of liquifying the area. Finally, there is a building up of a callus that eventually disappears as the bone grows into place where the fracture occurred. When the entire procedure is finished, there is often no scar at all, and one cannot tell the difference between that part of the bone and a portion that was never injured.

It was this knowledge, and the awareness that the salamander normally can regrow an extremity after amputation, that led Dr. Robert Becker, of the Upstate Medical Center of the State University of New York, to set out to determine why. That was two decades ago, and Becker has since published his findings, which include a theory on local regeneration of tissue. Using low-amperage electrical input, Becker was able to regrow extremities in frogs, and later in rats. He has worked with injured hearts in rats, and he postulates that regeneration of tissue in man will be happening almost routinely by the turn of the century. Work similar to Becker's is going on in laboratories all over the United States now and promises much in the way of results.

What about regeneration without external stimulation by electricity? The concepts of healing found in the Cayce readings would say that it is possible, for there is activity of the nervous system in man at the very low levels of amperage. The question arises—could thoughts be controlled to produce the optimal conditions for regrowth? Required would be an awareness within the body of its divine origin and the presence of what Cayce call God Forces within the very cells themselves that are concerned with regeneration. He commented:

For all healing—mental and material—is attuning each atom of the body, each reflex of the brain to an awareness of the Divine which lies within each cell.

3384–2

Know that all healing forces are within, not without! The applications from without are merely to create within a coordinating mental and spiritual force.

1196–7

Remember, the body does gradually renew itself constantly. Do not look upon the conditions which have existed as not being able to be eradicated from the system. Hold to that KNOWLEDGE—and don't think of it as just therapy—that the body CAN, the body DOES, renew itself!

1548–3

Healing, then—in the context of the Cayce material—is certainly an adventure in consciousness both for the doctor and for the patient; and a healing of the whole person becomes a responsible action for both parties involved in the process. Perhaps this idea is one of the concepts being born in the world today, as man moves into a new age of consciousness.

Chapter Four
REGENERATION AND LONGEVITY

Regeneration and longevity are a reality that can occur within one's own individual life. We are now about to survey the possibility of a long life and what may be required to accomplish such a goal. Further, such a goal implies that one will maintain a high degree of health and awareness, and if that awareness is related to the spiritual nature of man and is life-related, it becomes even more worthwhile.

Health and long life have a great deal to do with the electrical currents that course through the nervous system and the tissues of the body. Health and long life also bring us into direct contact with the idea of consciousness and face to face with the need for obeying the law of cycles that operate within our bodies. Regeneration itself is the constant rebuilding of the body through the division of cells and the ability of the body to restore to normal various parts that have lost their viability. Applied properly, the concepts of healing that have already been discussed will move one toward a lengthened life and a heightened state of awareness. However, there is more to be understood, if we are to more fully utilize the information in the Cayce material.

First, we must understand and apply the concept of consciousness. Consciousness, according to Cayce, differs in some manner from most definitions. I remember an instance in which someone asked the sleeping Cayce whether he should take castor oil for his present condition. Cayce, with his psychic-tongue in cheek, replied, "If you have a castor oil consciousness, take castor oil." I have often applied that concept in my practice of medicine, for many of my patients have a penicillin consciousness, and they need that drug. In their minds, they will not get well on the time schedule that they have set unless they take penicillin. So I administer penicillin, for we need to establish communication at some level, and it is my job to discern that level . . . if I am capable of it.

Cayce talked about consciousness in the cells of the body—even in the atom. Each part of our body, even each atom, has its job to do. Yet, as Cayce put it, we would not want the cells of the fingernail bed to start producing nasal tissue, nor vice versa. Each cell knows what it is supposed to do and does it; and each cell contributes to the total consciousness of our being.

One of the really challenging concepts found in the Cayce readings is that these very cells of the body may be completely unaware of their destiny, or, on the other hand, they may be completely "enlight-

ened." Perhaps one's growth in consciousness is related to the gradual awakening process that comes
about in these individual, unaware cells. If in a holistic sense this concept is valid, then is there not a
dominance in the direction or actions of an individual that is determined by the balance of power inside the body between the "aware" and the "unaware"
groups of cells?

Possibly our individual actions are more often dic-
tated by the "vote" that is taken among these cells,
rather than by our election to act as our minds
would tell us is the most creative way to go. The
latter way involves a will that is above the consciousness of the cells and an ability of the mind that is
part of the divine to discern what is creative. According to Cayce, such possibilities do exist.

Consciousness must also exist at an unconscious
level. This seems to be a contradiction, but it really
is not, since consciousness is simply awareness, and
we are always aware in some manner, even when we
sleep and dream. Cayce himself was certainly aware
of many things even when he was fully within his
own particular state of extended consciousness. Perhaps we should say that unconscious consciousness
is extended consciousness.

Within the consciousness of our bodies is the recognition of the importance of cycles. There is the
larger cycle of rebirth, which brings the good and
the bad, the constructive and the destructive, influences into our bodies. We also find the seven-year
cycle, in which, according to some medical sources
and certainly from the standpoint of the Cayce
readings, one completely changes every atom in his
body during that period of time.

There is the monthly menstrual cycle, which appears to be under the direction of the pineal gland
but which is certainly ruled to some extent by the
moon. Then there is the daily diurnal cycle, which
gives us trouble when we travel any great distance
east or west. These cycles are strong within our
bodies and play a part in every human life.

The importance of taking medications (or vitamins)
in a cyclic manner was emphasized again and again

in the readings. One of the most frequent bits of advice given by Cayce to those attempting to regain their health was to do the prescribed activity consistently and at the same time of day, if at all possible. Cayce often said that the body itself rebelled if something was started and then discontinued. Meditation also was to be accomplished at the same time of day.

Biological Rhythms in Human and Animal Physiology, an excellent publication of the National Institute of Mental Health, by Gay Gaer Luce, provides numerous examples of the importance of cycles. For example:

*Amphetamine injected in a certain dosage into rats during one portion of their daily activity cycle killed 6% of them; while injected in the same dosage during another point in their daily activity cycle, the fatality rate was 77%!

*Because of variations in the rhythm of amino acids, people who want to lose weight are advised to eat their heaviest meal in the morning.

*For those who travel great distances east or west by jet, or who shift day and night schedules for any reason, evidence exists that it takes three to five weeks before their various bodily cycles are coordinated again in their functioning.

Turning from cycles and a consideration of consciousness, we should ask, "What, really, does it mean to live a long time?" Edgar Cayce's response to such a question would undoubtedly be that, first, we contribute most to our length or shortness of days by our own concept of how long we *should* live. We must be productive, doing something toward meeting our individual purpose in life, contributing something to the world, or we lose our desire to stay here . . . and we die.

Some years ago a "Normative Aging Study" by the Veterans Administration forecast a normal life expectancy for the average American of 120–140 years. At about the same time this report was published in

1973, there appeared a newspaper story about Charlie Smith, who was celebrating his 131st birthday in Bartow, Florida. Charlie was at that time the oldest man in the United States drawing Social Security payments. He was described as not wearing glasses, hearing well, and liking to talk.

Then there was Shirali Mislimov, who at 168 years of age was still caring for his orchard, riding his horse, taking an active part in village politics in Russia, and whose young wife was only 106. It was only about two years after Shirali became famous for being the oldest person in the world that he suddenly died. It was almost as if he suddenly found out that, of all the people in the world, he was the oldest, and therefore the most likely person to go next . . . and he went.

We all want to live a long time, it would seem, *if* we can be vigorous and relatively healthy in the process and have our minds clear. All valid information points toward the concept that if the mind is kept active in creative matters, it will continue to function with the passage of years. Cayce readings substantiate this idea. From Russia and other parts of the world, we find that there are people who have lived far beyond the traditional three score and ten, proving beyond a doubt that it is *possible* to do so. Whether we can catch hold of the formula for doing so is another question.

The secret? Edgar Cayce implied that all knowledge is available within, if we seek patiently, persistently, and consistently. In discussing longevity, the Cayce readings speak of sources of life, destiny, origin, and the varying manifestations of life energy.

Cayce saw man as the greatest creation in the universe, created as a spiritual being with Godlike qualities and potential, manifesting as a seemingly physical being in this three-dimensional sphere, with consciousness dominating our nature, and with an overriding purpose and ideal often controlling even the length of our life span on Earth. This spiritual being maintains life and identity beyond what we call death, as it returns to the dimension of its origin, and can return again and again to the Earth plane, for learning and experience and growth of awareness.

The purpose, then, is not just to live a long time, but *to live*, for whatever length of time one is here, *so that the soul purpose is more fulfilled* as a result of the living. Cayce said many times what the sages and prophets throughout the ages have maintained as truth: that the quality of living—patience, kindness, forgiveness, understanding—is the goal, rather than the quantity. So, it is *how* one lives, rather than *how long*, that counts.

Cayce once gave the following selection from a reading to a man in his early forties:

> For there is every infusion within a normal body to replenish itself. And if there will be gained that consciousness, there need not be ever the necessity of a physical organism aging—other than that as is of the nominal desire of a body to give away to the surrounding forces or for its own rest.
>
> 1299—1

What, then, is to "give away to the surrounding forces"? Perhaps it is to succumb to the pressure of tensions that arise in the normal affairs of the day or to the unusual events that come into everyone's life. It is quite a job, it seems to me, to keep the kind of composure that will allow one to ride out all the events of the world and its activities today with that kind of equanimity.

The aging or leaving of the body "for its own rest" is a lot more understandable, and we see this nearly every day. When one partner passes through the door we call death, the spouse who is left might find that the need for rest is more than the body itself can stand, and he or she will pass on to the other side quite soon after.

Scientists tracking down the fountain of youth have discovered that their efforts can best be expended working with the endocrine and the immunological systems. In their study of the aging process, they have collectively come to the conclusion that body organs do not deteriorate dramatically with age

. . . neither the brain, the level of testosterone, the
healthy heart, nor the liver. Rather, they feel that
the Churchills and the Adenauers performed so well
at an advanced age because they were blessed generi-
cally with endocrine systems that stayed in balance
and immune systems that remained strong. From
the perspective of Edgar Cayce, however, these two
systems and their health are the product of emotions that are constructive, thoughts that are building in their nature, and an ideal and goal in life that
has spiritual foundations over the eons of time, space,
and patience.

In understanding the seven endocrine or spiritual-
glandular centers of the body, the thymus gland is
spoken of as the heart center or the love center. In
recent years, much research has identified that gland
as the master gland directing the immune forces of
the body in all their activities. Thymosin is a hormone produced by the thymus gland and has been
directly related to the aging process by the University of Texas medical researchers. Apparently, thymosin is directly related to immunity, and injecting
this hormone into mice increases their immunity
and resistance to disease. It has been known for
some time that cells from the thymus migrate to
other portions of the body and become centers of
lymphatic activity . . . among the most noteworthy
are the Peyer's patches.

The interesting correlation here with the Cayce
material is that Cayce attributed much importance
to the Peyer's patches—a series of aggregated lymph
nodules in the lining of the small intestine. According to Cayce, these patches tended to lessen in number as the body weakened. He suggested that regular
use of castor oil packs would tend to rejuvenate
these glands and thus be a major factor in the rejuvenation of the entire body. Drawing further from the
Cayce readings, one might say that the lack of
tensions, or the ability to handle them properly, a
strong faith that is evidenced by one's life, or a life
that is marked by regular prayer and meditation,
could be directly related to the number of Peyer's

patches present in one's body, which, in turn, could well have a strong influence on how long one lives.

Rebuilding the Peyer's patches is in essence a regeneration process, as is the rebuilding of the nervous system, and both lead to longevity and health. An article dealing with brain regeneration (*Medical World News*, July 21, 1972) led off with the following paragraph:

> Medical tradition has regarded the mature brain as static, changing only through disease, damage or senility. That picture is rapidly changing. New evidence presents a dynamic master organ—able to grow new pathways, repair damage, perhaps even accept a nerve transplant.

Cayce indicated in his readings that neurological conditions could be corrected, and that diseases such as multiple sclerosis could be cleared up, thereby implying that nervous tissue, myelin sheaths and the like, can actually regenerate, restoring the body to complete newness and perfect physical condition. This was never pictured as being a simple or an easy accomplishment, but the possibility was there. In other words, the brain could be rewired.

In the process of producing a state of longevity in any body, however, the regeneration or rejuvenation activity is not limited to the thymic system or to the nervous system. All parts of the body have this capability, and perhaps more so than we are willing to admit to ourselves. We find ourselves programmed by our environmental way of thinking, and probably by many lifetimes, in which we have been convinced that fifty, sixty, or seventy years are about all one should survive in the physical body.

Cayce, as well as most sensitives and parapsychologists, may have been considered for years to be "way out," but times are changing. Scientific investigations are beginning to give evidence that truth may indeed be gained by the human mind long before we figure it out and prove it by the painstaking, laborious, and *important* methodology of the scientist.

Chapter Five
HOLISTIC HEALTH AND SELF-CARE

A new direction in health care, called by some the self-care movement, is gaining more and more adherents. Dr. Lowell Levin, Yale University professor in the School of Public Health, has advocated health promotion activities by the lay person as a major movement of the future. Discussing the manner in which the average person may perform tasks related to his health and welfare, Dr. Levin pointed out that presently the housewife uses the thermometer, the blood pressure cuff, and the toothbrush (as well as the aspirin bottle, the mercurochrome, plain soap and water, and the healing touch). As responsibility is handed or delegated back to the patient for his or her own health, it will then be possible for physicians to be used "more parsimoniously, more precisely and more effectively." (*Arizona Health*, July 1977)

I recall how Dr. Art Ulene, a gynecologist on the West Coast, told a group of us several years ago that we should "give the body back to its rightful owner." This is the sort of statement that is suggested in the Cayce readings by implication, and it is the byword of the movement that is called holistic healing or holistic health. It is encouraging that professors and those in positions of leadership within medicine are beginning to recognize and teach what many practitioners have recognized for years: the patient needs to be part of the healing process. However, he can be a part of the process only if he is given responsibility and authority for such a role, and if he accepts the accountability for what takes place.

Edgar Cayce was ahead of his time during the early half of this century, when he gave more than fourteen thousand readings. He saw man consistently as a whole being—body, mind, and spirit. His suggestions for healing the body with a pill, a castor oil pack, a laying on of hands, a prayer, or with the surgeon's knife, were nearly always interspersed with comments directing the individual to recognize his spiritual origin and his spiritual destiny. His implication was that every event in one's life, whether an experience in human relationships or an illness of the human body, was truly an adventure in consciousness and would lead one, if willing to be led, into a more holistic state of being.

Health is a dynamic process, not a structure or a state to be arrived at. It must be sought after, and it must be maintained, for it involves the coordinating functions of all the organs and systems of the human body. It requires proper assimilation. It insists on adequate eliminations, and the circulatory system is vital to its attainment. We do not achieve health through the injection of an antibiotic or through an operation. We simply remove the insult that has been threatening the life of the body, and allow homeostasis of the body to once more be achieved—even though that level of bodily functioning may be far below what we would define as health. Health is traditionally defined as a state of perfect balance; and healing is that which brings about that kind of balance once again.

On the self-care side of health, there is a holistic approach formulated by doctors who have spent much of their lives seeking first spiritually. In 1978, Herbert Puryear, a clinical psychologist and an authority on the Edgar Cayce material, keynoted a symposium by defining a holistic lifestyle as follows:

1. A balance between the inner and the outer aspects of life.
2. A balance between the physical, mental, and spiritual portions of one's being.
3. Observe the cycles of life. Rejoice in the timing— things are brought forth in due season. Fulfill the purposes of the cycles of our own bodies, of our energies, of life itself.

4. The way of the middle path. Neither Jesus nor Buddha was an extremist. Rejoicing in the middle path shows our acceptance of the nature of things as they exist, of the values of the midpoint, and of our willingness to give up our tendencies to express the extremes in our actions.
5. There must be an ideal, a center, a place to which we may return. We must know what we believe, in Whom we believe, and in the centeredness of our own lives.

To further clarify developments in the self-care movement and what has been called holistic care, it should be mentioned that a movement was begun within the medical profession in 1978 that holds considerable promise for such care in the future. I am referring to the American Holistic Medical Association, which within nine months had a membership of over four hundred medical and osteopathic physicians. The principles of ethics of this organization speak directly to our discussion:

THE FIRST PRINCIPLE: The physician should render service to humanity with the full respect for the dignity of mankind in general and the total individual in particular. Physicians should consider total needs of patients, directing treatment toward the total person: body, mind and spirit. The treatment shall at all times be in the best interests of the patient.

ANOTHER PRINCIPLE: Physicians should recognize that patients have an inalienable right to share in making decisions pertaining to their treatment. The physicians should guide and educate their patients toward this goal and actively encourage patients to share in the responsibility for their care.

As I reflect on these signs of the times and on the situation in the world today, I realize we are in an age of major conceptual change, and in a world that is seeking its evolution toward the real goals that mankind has cherished for ages . . . and I sense the goodness that is coming about in the mind of man.

Chapter Six
SOME INDIVIDUAL RESEARCH

Edgar Cayce always said: "Try these things out, research them yourself, then write about them." The research comes first, the enlightenment afterward, and so the name of his own organization was derived—the Association for Research and Enlightenment (A.R.E.).

A case in point was shared with me by an A.R.E. member from West Palm Beach. Our researcher's interest had been stimulated by a Cayce reading that appeared in a booklet on gems and stones:

> Do not take this as being a thing of superstition or as something which would be a good luck charm, but if the entity will wear about its person, or in its pocket, a metal that is carbon steel—preferably in the groin pocket—it will prevent, it will ionize the body—by its very vibrations—to resist cold, congestion, and those inclinations for disturbance in the mucous membranes of the throat and nasal passages.
>
> 1842—1

After digesting this information, at least partially, our researcher decided to do something about it. He glued a piece of tool steel to a key so that he could carry it on his key chain in his pocket. He found it worked time and time again. At times, he reports, he feels a cold coming on—a tickle in the throat or nose—but it lasts only a couple of hours and then disappears. He no longer has any fear of being near someone who has a cold or flu.

Research at the personal level will never carry the impact on the scientist or the investigator of work done at the university level, but it has its own value. One such value is the realization by the individual that something real has happened within his own experience, and he has produced data that is meaningful and often helpful to other people, once this data is shared.

An interesting example was shared with me by a correspondent from the Midwest. This individual had found that he was afflicted recurrently with acute tonsilitis. He began using castor oil packs around his throat and found that one treatment, for one hour, produced excellent results. Five times he did this, and now, for the past five and a half years, he has had no recurrence of the tonsil infection.

Being an enterprising soul, as well as an A.R.E. member, he sought out a niece and a friend, both of whom had laryngitis, and suggested this kind of treatment. His results? Excellent! Finally, his wife developed a uterine infection that became the object of further research. Three times he had her apply a castor oil pack to her lower abdomen for an hour to an hour and a half. His results? The same. Perhaps his enthusiasm colored his results a bit, but perhaps his desire for results aided that healing energy that one does not always find readily available. Whatever the full story, whether it be the castor oil plant and its oil, the pure desire for healing, or the vibratory healing quality generated by our correspondent, the result, in the eyes of the individuals involved, was healing of the human body; and isn't that what it's all about?

Over the years, we have come to the conclusion that an approach to healing that might be called multilevel in its nature has had the greatest value to our patients. The problems a patient presents lead the physician to utilize several avenues of therapy directed, for the most part, toward upgrading the functions of the body that currently are not performing at their norm. A diet to improve the assimilation; a series of massages to mobilize the lymphatics toward better activity; these, plus other measures, often help a patient to a state of better health.

Approaching the restoration of health from this point of view is not limited, however, to the physician.

One of our Clinic doctors received a letter from a correspondent who had done the same thing for herself:

> I am now free of the pains I have had in my neck and back for the last five years! The pain was suddenly gone several weeks ago and has not returned. I no longer need to take any muscle relaxants or pain pills. I don't have to tell you what a miracle this is for me! . . . I feel I owe my recovery to three factors:
>
> 1. I have applied the castor oil packs to my abdomen and back daily for almost six months;
>
> 2. My attitude about my sickness and my life in general has radically changed for the better since I was introduced to the Edgar Cayce philosophy; and
>
> 3. Many people, like you, have been praying for me.

Physical assistance, changes in mental attitude ("Mind is the builder!"), and spiritual help: it is difficult to resist therapy like that.

In nearly twenty years of association with the concepts of healing and regeneration found in the Cayce readings, my experience and my mind tell me that all people should have at least the opportunity to bring about healing in their own body or in aiding another. This can be done by prayer, of course, which is usually not dramatic, even though it is effective. Utilizing the same concept that all healing comes from within the body, the opportunity might come through the application of a castor oil pack or vinegar and salt, or some such remedy that often is not only dramatic in its effectiveness but also satisfies that *desire for healing*. The experience of a Kansas City woman is a case in point:

> First, believe me, when it comes to my children's health, I am not in the least likely to take chances, so do not think I acted impulsively or took any

unusual chances. It started on a Sunday morning when my five-year-old complained that his foot hurt and he had some red streaks on his ankle. I took his temperature, and it was normal, but where he had stepped on a nail the previous day, it was now quite red, and there were two or three streaks raised like welts, almost to his knee. I had never seen blood-poisoning streaks before, but I was sure that it was blood poisoning, but my husband didn't think so.

Being Sunday morning, the prospect of a trip to the hospital emergency room wasn't pleasing. I thought I would try the Cayce castor oil packs and heat and would give it no longer than four hours. If he was running a temperature or was worse in any way by that time, I would call the doctor. I had used the packs for bruises and swelling but never for anything really serious before. I put the pack on and wrapped an elastic bandage around it, then fastened the heating pad around that and made him sit and keep his foot elevated. At the end of four hours, the red streaks were definitely fading and the swelling had disappeared. The pain was nearly gone also, and there was no temperature elevation. I left the pack on with heat the rest of the day, then that night took off the heating pad, leaving the pack in place.

By the next morning, the foot looked completely normal, and when my boy stepped on it, there was no pain. I watched him carefully for several days, but the symptoms never came back, and everything was great. No shots or pills and no doctor bill, or hospital bill, and it cleared up so fast. I have since used it for the same type of infection with the same results.

It's a funny thing, though. In working with my kids, the ones that believe it will help are helped. The one daughter that does not believe in home remedies and faith healing was not helped.

Chapter Seven
SOME SUMMARY OBSERVATIONS

We have described health and healing in a variety of ways. The Edgar Cayce material seems to be saying that any therapy that proposes to heal the body must make the vibrations of the body come into harmony or equilibrium with the vibrations of the physical plane in which we live.

Healing of the body is often like the well-known "stitch in time" that saved nine; or it might be like the finger in the dike. In the first instance, it produced a whole cloth once again; in the latter, a solid wall against the water that threatened flooding. More and more, it seems to me that the healing process really is often a single move to restore a balance to the human body.

Healing is often a mystery even to the physician. There are nearly nine thousand readings in Virginia Beach dealing in one manner or another with the philosophy of healing, as well as with the manners, means, and reasons involved in restoring the body to normal. Cayce seemed to dwell on the spiritual quality more than any other factor as he discoursed on the healing process and how it should be brought into action. Also, he talked more about persistence than any of the other spiritual qualities. Someone has said that neither talent nor genius nor education allow one to succeed with certainty; but persistence combined with determination—a combination of patience and consistency—just cannot be denied. It works in all facets of life and most certainly in the healing of the body.

Physiological rehabilitation is a term we have given to our own kind of treatment designed to regenerate tissue and bring healing to our patients. Healing in any manner, of course, is still healing, and the result is a healthy, normal human body. Perhaps it

would be more accurate to say a *healthier* body.
Rehabilitation in this manner is not simply the restoration of the muscular structure and coordination;
rather, it is the regeneration of the cellular structure
and the function of nerve, glandular, and organic
tissues. These being aided, the entire physical organism then functions at a more normal level.

Patience in the healing process is a necessity, especially when a long-standing problem of the body is
in the various stages of dissolution, or when one
has suffered with a problem over a long period of
time. When the patient is young and has not experienced many years of life with its vicissitudes, it is
more difficult, I think, to accept a long-term therapy
program, and the inevitable question arises: "How
long will I need to continue this therapy program?"
The sleeping Cayce addressed this question when
faced with a problem of vitiligo:

> Q = 11: Can you specify the length of time it will
> take before the spots disappear entirely?
>
> A = 11: How long before tomorrow? How long be-
> fore or since yesterday? These are a matter of the
> mental concept. If it is the desire, then work to-
> wards it. But is the desire for the outlook or for
> the actual conditions? Is it of a spiritual or purely
> material nature? Study this that you are asking,
> and know that the sources consider not time.
>
>   1490–4

Throughout the Cayce readings is the recurrent
theme that all healing comes from one source,
whether it is by a prayer, a pill, a surgical knife, or
an electrical treatment . . . be it high vibration or
low vibration in type. Many who read the Cayce
material think erroneously that medicine, surgery,
and X-ray have no place in the regimen suggested by
this unconscious psychic source. The fact is that
these treatments, which can and do bring healing to
the body, are numbered among those found in the
readings. However, like any treatments, they need to
be used in the right manner and with the proper

goals in mind—the healing of the body or the bringing to the body its normal forces of vitality and life.
A case in point was when Cayce suggested surgery
for his own physical body; an appendectomy that
the attending physicians did not think was necessary.
As it turned out, it was; and, in the process, it was
discovered that the appendix was practically ruptured!

Healing of any nature comes about in different
ways in different individuals. A host of methods
exists to restore the body to its normal functioning.
I believe it is always important to keep this concept
uppermost in our minds. For, as we have indicated,
the restoration of normal function is the real healing
of the body, and real healing is directly connected to
consciousness:

> For all healing comes from the one source. And
> whether there is the application of foods, exercise,
> medicine, or even the knife—it is to bring [to] the
> consciousness of the forces within the body, that
> aid in reproducing themselves [which is] the aware-
> ness of creative or God forces.
>
> 2962–1

The suggestions in the Cayce material were given
by a man in touch with Universal Forces. They are
fashioned so that people with little knowledge of
their own bodies can begin to utilize the information on themselves. It not only saves money, but it
helps our nation with a major problem facing us at
the present time—the problem of health care delivery.
The more effectively people can learn to stay healthy
and cure their own minor (and sometimes not-so-
minor) ailments, the fewer physicians and health
care facilities will be needed.

Healing of the body seems to be a universal human need. In the Bible, Jesus related healing to
forgiveness of sin, but today we are chary in our
attitude toward sin. We hesitate to commit it, and
hesitate even more to define it. Cayce had no com-
punction about discussing the relationship between
sin and sickness. According to him: "Sickness is sin
lying at your own doorstep." He hastened to add

that, in his definition, sin was basically a life activity directed selfward rather than toward the service of others.

Service to others is the primary theme found in the Cayce readings and is the manner in which one finds a oneness with God. It is evident from those same readings that one's capacity to stray off the path in a given lifetime may not manifest its karma (the reaping of what one has sown) until the next lifetime, or the next, or the next. It often leaves us puzzled when we see someone ill or suffering for no apparent reason, until we look at the picture in perspective—until we see the individual as being active in several lifetimes, not just one.

Jesus, when he healed one man, said: "Go, and sin no more." We might add to that by saying to ourselves, "Physician, heal thyself!" Cayce's vocabulary moved effortlessly from the physical to the metaphysical, and he seemed always to be saying the same thing in different terms. He saw a oneness of the body, a oneness of all beings, and a oneness of God and man.

Part Two
TAKING ACTION

Chapter Eight
YOU CAN DO IT

Throughout my thirty-five years of medical training and experience, I have been impressed by the number of people who appear to get well spontaneously. These spontaneous recoveries are not really cloaked in mystery, however, if we place them in the context of information discussed earlier in this book. There are functions of the body that repulse disease and bring rejuvenation. The *life factor* is always ready to be utilized; we have but to recognize that it exists and to call upon it, in one form or another.

Perhaps those cures that we call spontaneous are really the result of the afflicted person, or one close to him, applying to the mind, the spirit, or the body a simple procedure that reverses things inside, and health begins its trip back home to the body. The role of the mind in the healing process today cannot be denied. It is undoubtedly important for every chronically ill person to recognize *with his mind* where he is in relationship to health in order that the true healing process may go forward.

Individuals who are ill are often in rebellion against that which brought about the illness, failing to recognize that the origin of their problem does not lie elsewhere than at their own doorstep. Their rebellion, their warfare, is truly within their own bodies. They must let go of the rebellion before the trek back to peace is begun—and the healing process begins. It is always a fascinating story when one comes into that awareness that he should in reality accept himself and begin working from a new level of consciousness. Most of the time we are not able to see the mental block in our consciousness that is denying to us the healing process, and thus we don't get well. Perhaps we learn the lesson then through the sickness. But we *can* recognize the block if we do a bit of understanding relative to our makeup.

A single sentence from a Cayce reading may help us on this score, as we explore its rather far-reaching ramifications.

> Then there is the mental body, accredited oft with activity from reflexes or impulses of the nervous systems of the individual.
>
> 2402–1

Cayce had just discussed the physical body and went on to talk about the soul body. But the mental body was given a cloak of mystery. Cayce seemed to be saying that the mind—which is the builder—is often given the credit for thinking, for acting in a creative manner, when in reality it is just reacting reflexively from patterns of habit, of energy, and of electricity created by that same individual in his nervous system.

It's sort of like when I use a reflex hammer to elicit a patellar reflex on the knee of a patient sitting on the examining table. The leg suddenly kicks upward, and often the patient will laugh and say, "Look at that, would you—that leg kicks up all by itself."

The mind works through the nervous system, and we necessarily create many habitual responses. It would be difficult to live normally without these habits. But there are not only the physical body responses; there are the mental patterns that are created by our environment, such as our religious beliefs, our political tendencies, our ways of spending or keeping or giving money. These and other neurological patterns become part of "the way I am!" Or at least we say so. Thus, when one faces a situation where mental activity is required, one is very likely to tune in his thought processes to patterns he has already created, through experiences in lifetimes past and present, and he reacts rather than acts. It would be helpful, then, if we looked at our mind's decision much like the patient looking at his leg, and we said, "Look at that, would you, that mind kicked up all by itself!"

Indeed, the mind is often credited with activity when it is only a reflex or an impulse from the cerebrospinal or the autonomic nervous system. However, *the creative mind* must go past these barriers of electroneurological patterns and reach the freedom of true thought before most of the problems of this world can be solved. And certainly this must be accomplished by those who are seeking their own individual spontaneous remission. The clear, creative mind must be active, and the body must then take action in accord with the thought. With this in mind, let us examine the processes of visualization and suggestion—processes of the mind that enable the body to take action.

Visualization and Sugggestion

Visualization is really speaking to the unconscious mind in its own language. The unconscious mind dwells in the autonomic nervous system and its centers of control, and it gives us messages through pictures and symbols. Dreams are evidence of this. It has gradually been understood that the unconscious will not take orders from the higher mind unless these orders come in the symbolic language of the unconscious, and unless the message gets through without being garbled. If we say to the stomach, "Quit producing so much harmful acid!" the stomach will not obey, although our higher mind really has the right to request—or even demand—such an action on the part of the stomach.

However, if we were to allow our bodies to become thoroughly relaxed—perhaps with music like Barber's "Adagio for Strings" playing in the background—and then we visualized, with our minds, a valley out in the country, where raging waters had cut furrows in the ground and little vegetation had been able to grow, we would be starting the process of speaking to the autonomic nervous system. We would be telling the unconscious that our stomach is like that valley. The unconscious would understand, and undoubtedly would agree. Then we would need to visualize the sun coming out, the storm clouds clearing up, and peace returning to the valley; the grass begins to grow and the vegetation begins to heal the furrows in the earth.

Through such symbolic communication we bridge the gap between the conscious and the unconscious. With the assistance of music and relaxation, we stand ready to see beneficial things happening to our stomach.

Cayce was ahead of his time with this method of healing. Reading what he had to say about it helps to convey an understanding of the process and to give depth to the idea. For example:

Q-3: Any spiritual advice for this body?

A-3: The body is spiritual in its aspects and its reaction. If the body will aid self in those applications as may be made for same, *see* self—in the periods when the body enters into the quiet—*healed* as it, the body, *would* be healed. *Vision* self *being* aided by those applications. Know what each application is for, *seeing* that *doing* that within self. Keep the mind in that attitude as makes for *continuity* of forces manifesting through self—a continual flow, see?

326-1

Those vibrations as may be had by the concerted activity of individuals, that may be able to raise their *own* imaginative (if so chosen to be called) forces within self, to see those activities taking place within the active forces of the body, [5576], we will find this will also aid. *Seek* and ye shall find; *knock* and it will be opened! *See* that being accomplished, and it will aid much.

5576-1

So, the mind should be used creatively in many ways as we learn how to bring healing to our own bodies. The mind truly is the builder—of all our distresses, certainly, but also of our health and our rejuvenation and whatever longevity we are willing to settle for.

Some years ago, a friend told me how she had slipped in the kitchen, and in reaching out to keep herself from falling, she pressed the back of her right hand against a red-hot burner on her stove. It sizzled. My friend believes in the healing power of the mind, but she put her hand in cold water anyway. She refused to look at it, although her husband didn't like the way her fingers looked. It was bedtime, and she placed her hand in ice water at her bedside. After a bit, she said, she realized that faith in the healing power was not consistent with ice water, so she chose the former, letting the ice treatment go by the boards. She used no bandage and she slept well. In the morning, there was only a very slight trace of a scar where the burn had been.

And then there is the story that osteopathic psychiatrist Fred Martin related to me about a patient's injured knee and its resolution. The therapy he used is strikingly similar to the visualization process:

> After the third visit with an outpatient in psychotherapy, she slipped on the ice and fell, twisting her right knee . . . X-rays by the family doctor were reported as negative by her when she limped into my office one week after the injury. (I had been seeing her twice a week.) The knee was obviously swollen with a moderate-sized hematoma visible on the medial aspect of the knee. She walked on her right toes with the knee flexed about fifteen to twenty degrees and sat with the knee flexed the same way. During the hour, nothing was said about the knee until at the end I told her that I had a few suggestions which might help her knee. She was willing. She was mentally in what I call a "mood of relaxation," which has some similarities to a light state of hypnosis. In this mood, ego syntonic suggestions are fairly well accepted, but the critical faculty of the ego is fully functioning. Using some ideas that I had developed from the readings, I suggested that a field of healing energy in tune with the universal creative forces could develop around her hip, thigh, and down past her knee and that the energy field

would just sort of suspend all the tissues so that the swelling could rapidly flow out, new fluids and blood flow through, and the nerves that were irritated quiet down and supply the guiding impulses needed for healing. I further suggested that this process would reestablish the normal balance of forces within the injured tissues and with the entire body and that the process could take place at a remarkably rapid rate. The energy field was to remain present until healing had been complete.

Next visit [four days later] . . . the knee was "well." There was no swelling, no pain, and the discoloration was completely gone—cleared overnight. . . . She has not complained about the knee since.

Fred told me not only that had she no limp and no real problems with the knee, but that the very next morning after the suggestions had been given, her symptoms were gone.

Planning the Process of Healing

Not only must we use our creative minds in healing ourselves, but we must play a lead role in planning the process of healing. There are numerous methods that can be applied to any situation, aside from the mind and from spiritual sources. These are the practical, down-to-earth methods of healing the physical body, and the major part of this book is devoted to dealing with those methods, and especially with how they are applied to the body in the case of specific disease conditions or malfunctions of a physiological process.

A most obvious way of determining if one is ill is simply by recognizing a dis-ease within one's body or by having a complete physical examination and history in a physician's office. However, this approach frequently does not reflect the stresses of life that we experience, nor does it measure the toll that has been taken of the body by those stresses.

Changes in life are always stress-producing. It doesn't matter whether they are nice or nasty changes, whether we like them or hate to see them come about. Dr. Holmes of the Washington (state) Medical School devised a chart that measures the values of different events in the living experience and gives one a good estimate of how much the stresses of life are impinging on his level of good health. We use it routinely on all our full medical examinations to detect tendencies, for tendencies are perhaps even more important than exhibited illness. Tendencies can be corrected—much like going down the wrong turn-off when it is discovered early on that an error in direction has been made. We can always turn back and get on the right road again.

Health is a continuing process of change, and it is reasonable to note that positive, constructive habits of eating, sleeping, exercising, acting, thinking, and believing change the body for the better, while the reverse is also true. Stressful living is a way of eating, sleeping, exercising, acting, thinking, and believing that creates trouble for the human body. To measure the stresses, "good" or "bad," is to evaluate how much of this destructive activity is going on; and at the same time to give assistance in knowing when to change so that we do not continue traveling down a dead-end road. In addition to internal stresses, there are also stresses from outside.

At the University of Washington in Seattle, Thomas H. Holmes, M.D., developed the Social Readjustment Rating Scale. You will find this scale at the end of this chapter. In our Clinic, where we have used it for the past ten to fifteen years, we call it the Holmes Life Changes Chart. Dr. Holmes suggests that when you rate yourself against the chart for the past year, you can predict your tendency for health or sickness in the near future. With 150–299 life change units, you have about a fifty percent probability of getting sick in the near future; with less than 150 life change units, you have only about a thirty percent probability of getting sick in the near future.

Dr. Holmes offers the following suggestions for using the Social Readjustment Rating Scale to maintain health and prevent illness:

1. Become familiar with the life events and the amount of change they require.
2. Put the scale where you and the family can easily see it several times a day.
3. With practice you can recognize when a life event happens.
4. Think about the meaning of the event for you and try to identify some of the feelings you experience.
5. Think about the different ways you might best adjust to the event.
6. Take your time in arriving at decisions.
7. If possible, anticipate life changes and plan for them well in advance.
8. Pace yourself. It can be done even if you are in a hurry.
9. Look at the accomplishment of a task as part of daily living and avoid looking at such an achievement as a "stopping point" or a "time of letting down."

At the Clinic we use this information to tell our patients that a tendency exists, and that they can do something about it by creating more constructive activities in their lives: improvement of diet, more sleep, and more regular, reasonable exercise. With a bit of applied wisdom—recognizing that the mind is the builder—you can be your own health adviser. With some reevaluating and restructuring of your activities, you can take the steps necessary to maintain or improve your level of health. As Edgar Cayce would say, "Start where you are . . . take what you have in hand . . . and begin! Begin!" You can do it!

The Social Readjustment Rating Scale*

Life Event	Mean Value
1. Death of spouse	100
2. Divorce	73
3. Marital separation from mate	65
4. Detention in jail or other institution	63
5. Death of a close family member	63
6. Major personal injury or illness	53
7. Marriage	50
8. Being fired at work	47
9. Marital reconcilation with mate	45
10. Retirement from work	45
11. Major change in the health or behavior of a family member	44
12. Pregnancy	40
13. Sexual difficulties	39
14. Gaining a new family member (e.g., through birth, adoption, oldster moving in, etc.)	39
15. Major business readjustment (e.g., merger, reorganization, bankruptcy, etc.)	39
16. Major change in financial state (e.g., a lot worse off or a lot better off than usual)	38
17. Death of a close friend	37
18. Changing to a different line of work	36
19. Major change in the number of arguments with spouse (e.g., either a lot more or a lot less than usual regarding childrearing, personal habits, etc.)	35
20. Taking out a mortgage or loan for a major purchase (e.g., for a home, business, etc.)	31
21. Foreclosure on a mortgage or loan	30

*T. H. Holmes and R. H. Rahe, The Social Readjustment Rating Scale, *Journal of Psychosomatic Research* 11(1967): 213–18.

22. Major change in responsibilities at work (e.g., promotion, demotion, lateral transfer) 29
23. Son or daughter leaving home (e.g., marriage, attending college, etc.) 29
24. Trouble with in-laws 29
25. Outstanding personal achievement .. 28
26. Wife beginning or ceasing work outside the home 26
27. Beginning or ceasing formal schooling 26
28. Major change in living conditions (e.g., building a new home, remodeling, deterioration of home or neighborhood) 25
29. Revision of personal habits (dress, manners, association, etc.) 24
30. Troubles with the boss 23
31. Major change in working hours or conditions 20
32. Change in residence 20
33. Changing to a new school 20
34. Major change in usual type and/or amount of recreation 19
35. Major change in church activities (e.g., a lot more or a lot less than usual) 19
36. Major change in social activities (e.g., clubs, dancing, movies, visiting, etc.) 18
37. Taking out a mortgage or loan for a lesser purchase (e.g., for a car, TV, freezer, etc.) 17
38. Major change in sleeping habits (a lot more or a lot less sleep, or change in part of day when asleep) 16
39. Major change in number of family get-togethers (e.g., a lot more or a lot less than usual) 15
40. Major change in eating habits (a lot more or a lot less food intake, or very different meal hours or surroundings) 15

Life Event	Mean Value
41. Vacation	13
42. Christmas	12
43. Minor violations of the law (e.g., traffic tickets, jaywalking, disturbing the peace, etc.)	11

Chapter Nine
CASTOR OIL PACKS

In 1967, I wrote a book about the use of castor oil packs in the clinical practice of medicine. Eighty-one individual case studies were covered in the book. Of all the therapies I have used in my practice of medicine, I have never found any that surpasses castor oil in its usefulness, its healing qualities, and its scope of therapeutic application. I have used and recommended castor oil, in packs, local applications, drops, and large dosages by mouth, literally thousands of times, and only in two or three instances have I found a patient allergic or sensitive to it. Problems people have tackled with castor oil range from appendicitis to scleroderma, and include pain syndromes, slipped discs, hyperactivity, tumors, tinnitus, nausea, etc.

The Palma Christi—the Palm of Christ—is the name given during the Middle Ages to the common castor oil plant.* No one knows why, exactly, it was so named. But it's interesting to consider the importance of symbols and the place symbology plays in the lives of men on Earth. Was it just coincidence when our eight-year-old son, David, told us one morning when he awakened that he had had a dream that Jesus put his hand on his back, and his back got better? David had fallen severely on the sharp edge of a carpeted step just before going to bed, and we were apprehensive about a possible fracture of a

*William A. McGarey, M.D., *Edgar Cayce and the Palma Christi* (Virginia Beach: A.R.E. Press, 1967.)

vertebra. It hurt him so much that nothing helped but to keep him quiet. We placed a castor oil pack on the injured spot, and he slept on the floor beside us that night, very restless until about four o'clock, when suddenly he quieted down and slept soundly.

When he awoke and told us the dream, we examined his back. It was fully normal in all respects. There was no pain, no aching, no sign of injury. What caused the healing? Was it imagination? Was it the soothing only of the oil pack? Was it a vibratory effect? Was it a spiritual healing? Certainly my medical experience of more than twenty years at that point told me there *should* have been some very painful muscles and bones in the morning, at the very least. But there weren't. David traveled five hundred miles with us that day and was examined by the late Dr. Mayo Hotten. Mayo could find no evidence of any injury.

On another occasion, one of our boys stepped on a three-pronged metal hanger (used for pegboards) and punctured the sole of his foot rather deeply in two places. After the bleeding was stopped, a sloppy castor oil pack was applied and kept in place until healing was almost complete—a matter of just a few days. The pain was eased immediately upon application of the pack, and weight was put on the injured foot the second day. Healing progressed without event, and the time of healing was certainly decreased.

The healing abilities of the castor oil pack placed on the abdomen were indicated by an individual who wrote:

> I used the castor oil packs for a fibroid tumor on my uterus. I used the three thicknesses of flannel with the oil and a heating pad three or four nights a week. I started about 9:30 P.M. and would read until sleepy and turn out the lights and heating pad at the same time, leaving the flannel and heating pad in place, and I would sleep until I would be ready to turn over (about 1:00 A.M.) and then remove it all. This continued about six months. At my next yearly checkup the doctor said (the fibroid) had disappeared.

Another letter came to me some time ago from a woman who applied information on her own: "I thought you might be interested in hearing that my mother had a lump near her vagina. We applied castor oil and camphorated oil. In three weeks, it reduced in size from the size of a walnut to the size of a pea; in five weeks it was gone, and has not returned."

Recently a boy of about fifteen years of age appeared in my office on crutches about forty-eight hours after he had had a laceration of his right ankle sutured in an emergency room. It was a small laceration, about a half-inch long, but it hurt him so much that he could not put his weight on his foot. Thus, he had the crutches. I examined the wound. It was healing nicely, with no sign of infection. It was extremely tender to the touch, and I assumed that there had been involvement of nerve tissue to an undue degree, since there was no tendon involvement. The boy was instructed to keep a soft pad of cloth saturated with castor oil on the wound overnight for the next few nights, held in place with an elastic bandage. The pain was nearly gone in twenty-four hours, absent in forty-eight hours, and he was playing football (against orders) in seventy-two hours . . . before the sutures were removed.

It is always difficult to identify why these packs produce the effect that is so frequently seen. I've had patients tell me that the castor oil pack is better for them than the best tranquilizer they have ever taken. It seems to bring peace into the body in a way that is mysterious but effective. Perhaps that is why they are so effective in dispelling the disease syndromes to which we all are subject.

Why Does it Work?

One concept that helps me understand why these packs are helpful in such a wide variety of conditions is the nature of castor oil when it is taken internally. It is cleansing to the entire intestinal tract, and, by reason of the proximity of the blood and lymphatic streams to the intestinal lumen, it is also cleansing to these vital streams of fluid.

Lymph is a fluid similar to blood but lacking red blood cells. Lymph also has other characteristics that differentiate it from blood. It is more alkaline in nature than is the bloodstream. It also has its beginnings in the intercellular spaces of the body, gathering minute streams of lymph into larger streams, until—through the thoracic duct, primarily—the lymph is emptied into the venous channels in the mediastinum of the chest and becomes part of the blood. It acts as a cleanser of the individual cells, since the capillaries of the arterial stream cannot take some waste products and other manufactured portions of cellular activity back into their own vessels. And the lymph passes through the various lymph nodes, the walls of the intestines, the liver, and the Peyer's patches.

It appears, from clinical observation of the manner in which various conditions respond to the packs, that castor oil has the effect of stimulating the activity of the lymphatic streams while at the same time enhancing the elimination of toxic substances from the cells locally where the castor oil is applied.

When an area that has been injured, or is inflamed for one reason or another, is treated with the packs, the cellular tissue in that area is capable of responding more normally with toxins removed, and thus is able to take care of the infection or inflammation.

An example of this kind of activity came to my attention from a doctor whose son had smashed his hand between two rocks. There were no fractures, but the hand was "badly abraised and contused." She continued the story:

> Against my medical training and my husband's we applied a warm castor oil pack to the hand. The next morning the results were dramatic. The swelling had completely subsided and healing had occurred at an incredible rate. By the third day, healing was complete. . . . The remarkable thing other than the healing was the absence of pain after an hour following the application of the pack.

Stories adding evidence to the concept of lymphatic stimulation and cleansing action abound: A sore throat "suddenly evaporated in fifteen minutes in what felt like a rush of running water" after the pack was placed on the abdomen. Two large nodules on the vocal cord, diagnosed by laryngoscopy, causing hoarseness in a twelve-year-old boy, gradually disappeared over a three-month period, on a regimen of packs to the neck three days in a row, resting two days, and then repeating. A sebacious cyst of the chest wall spontaneously opened and healed after three weeks of daily application of castor oil. A much more important response followed an automobile accident and the diagnosis of a possible ruptured spleen. Surgery was withheld, castor oil packs were applied, and in four days the patient was discharged, the doctor giving the packs the credit.

In the early years of my using these packs, when I would suggest such a therapy, often the patient would say, "What in the world is a castor oil pack?" I would patiently explain, or try to do so, telling them that they were suggested by a psychic named Edgar Cayce, etc., etc. Usually the patient would leave in great wonderment, with a fifty-fifty chance of using the pack.

Finally, I had instruction sheets printed up on our letterhead, giving all the details of how to make a pack and how to use it. Then, when a patient would ask, "What in the world is a castor oil pack?" I would answer, "You mean you've never heard of a castor oil pack?" And with great wonderment in my voice and my face, I would hand him an instruction sheet. It was a great relief.

How to Make and Use a Castor Oil Pack

To make a castor oil pack, you will need the following materials:

1. Flannel cloth
2. Plastic sheet—medium thickness
3. Electric heating pad
4. Bath towel
5. Two safety pins

First, prepare a soft flannel cloth, preferably of wool flannel, but cotton flannel is all right if wool is not available. The cloth should be two to four thicknesses when folded, and should measure about ten inches in width and twelve to fourteen inches in length after it is folded. This is the size needed for abdominal application; other areas of the body would need whatever size pack seems applicable.

Next, pour some castor oil onto the cloth. This can be done without soiling, if a plastic sheet is placed underneath the cloth. Make sure the cloth is wet but not dripping with castor oil. Then apply the cloth to the area that needs the treatment.

Then apply a plastic covering over the soaked flannel cloth. On top of that place a heating pad and turn it up to "medium" to begin with—then to "high" if the body tolerates it. Finally, it will probably help you if you wrap a towel, folded lengthwise, around the entire area and fasten it with safety pins.

The pack should remain in place between one hour and one and a half hours. Then the skin should be cleansed with a baking-soda solution prepared by adding two teaspoons of baking soda to a quart of water.

The flannel pack need not be discarded after one application, but may be kept in a plastic container for future use. The recommended frequency for use of a castor oil pack can vary between one and seven consecutive days per week. Often it is also suggested to take tolerable amounts of olive oil after every third treatment.

What About Faith—Where Does it Fit in?

The physician is often faced with this very real question. And if he meets those moments of truth within himself, he also must ask about the real nature of healing. Just exactly what is it? And how does it come about? I recently received a letter from a person who probably does not really know what happened inside herself phenomenologically, but her case undoubtedly is one that demonstrates the place of faith in the healing process. And it brings to my mind also the statement that Cayce made once, describing how castor oil affected tissues in a manner to bring the spirit into closer communication with the material body. A strange statement, but here is what happened.

Our friend underwent surgery for a hiatus hernia last December and did poorly postoperatively, perhaps partly because hospital personnel went on strike the second day after her surgery. Her recovery was slow; she was glad to get back home; but she developed thrombophlebitis in the left forearm, which responded poorly to routine soaking. She was given a drug that brought on severe further complications.

> Within a week, I'd gained ten pounds, my face was bloated, I could neither urinate nor evacuate, so I was reluctant to put anything more into my system after a few days. My vision was still blurred, and there was no depth perception; it was difficult to find the center of a doorway in walking from room to room.

This was nearly eight weeks after the surgery, and just a few days after this problem, she woke one Monday morning with severe abdominal pain. After consulting with a friend who had used castor oil packs, she immediately started applying them on her abdomen. Twice that Monday she applied the packs.

> Tuesday I woke with a definite feeling of more comfort and improvement; applied packs for one and a half hours that evening.
>
> Wednesday morning I felt a more nearly complete comfort in the entire abdominal area, and again applied packs that night for one and a half hours.
>
> Thursday upon awakening, there was no distension or discomfort in any portion of the entire torso. After the usual two cups of tea, a quite satisfactory evacuation brought as much mental as physical comfort, followed two hours later by a complete relief.

She continued using the packs for four weeks more and progressed to full recovery. But perhaps the key to her success is found in the following extract of her letter:

> Each of the four evenings, while packs were in place, I read and reread portions of the *Palma Christi*, making certain I was in a positive and meditative frame of mind. I had, I do have, and I will ever continue to have an absolute confidence in the efficacy of the packs. . . .

Faith is part of the picture, isn't it? Perhaps this woman has a faith so deep that it raises those powers of healing that Cayce often mentioned. Perhaps she herself is a healer. If we can rely on what came through the Cayce material, then healing is a Divine influence, interjected into the atomic, electrical nature of the human being and his environment.

As an individual places faith in the healing power even of the castor oil packs, perhaps one could say "self brings those *little* things necessary . . . so does the *entity become* the healer." And the healing is a raising of atomic forces in a positive vibration and a breaking down of destructive forces—a material healing, done through Creative Forces, which are God in manifestation. Who or what does the healing? The doctor? The patient? The packs? The faith? Or is all healing perhaps a slightly different manifestation of an original power that we admittedly know little about?

The stories developing out of the use of these packs—whether or not faith is the strongest factor—are fascinating to me, because they seem to be telling me that there really is the ability in simple substances to enliven, to awaken the normal, healthy, vital capabilities within the tissues and consciousness of the body to bring about healing in the most unusual conditions of the body.

Strange substance, this oil from the seed of the *Ricinus communis!* One begins to understand why, in the Middle Ages, someone called this plant the Palm of Christ, the Palma Christi. In the Cayce readings, it was suggested only several times that it be given by mouth, rather than in the form of a pack applied to the body externally. But, like Cayce once said, "if you have a castor oil consciousness, take castor oil."

Chapter Ten
DIET AND NUTRITION

It is extremely important to the individual human being, when considering the foodstuffs he puts into his mouth, to choose those foods that are constructive for his own particular needs and that will be assimilated. The body does not live and flourish on what is eaten—rather, it takes life from what is digested, absorbed into the lymph and bloodstream, and then made part of the living, dividing, and growing cells of the body. This process is called assimilation, and many factors can divert what appears to be food into channels of elimination long before it can be utilized by the body tissues as energy to grow by.

In a recent 165-page supplement of the *Journal of the American Medical Association*, where there were literally hundreds of courses, programs, lectures, and seminars on subjects ranging from abortion to neurosurgery, the word *nutrition* was not mentioned even once. Without good nutrition to guide one's body growth, development, and health, one is also hampered in his thinking and in his development of a spiritually oriented life.

Yet, the message from the Edgar Cayce readings is that we are what we eat—as well as what we believe and think. There are probably hundreds of diets for various purposes suggested by the readings. It is our experience that any diet will be strongly influenced by the emotions, attitudes, and activities that accompany it. Thus, even when one eats the very best food for his body and has the potential to take this food through all the steps of assimilation, one's very attitudes can destroy the nutritional benefits by blocking assimilation; the food then literally goes to waste.

It is also our experience and understanding that *any* diet will be aided and perhaps corrected for a particular body by praying over the food before eating. Finally, we cannot forget the biblical injunction that, in the last analysis, it is more important what comes out of the mouth than what goes into it: for what goes into the mouth eventually passes through the body and is eliminated; but what comes out through the mouth from the heart, delivers good or evil and the corresponding constructive or destructive influences on the body.

In all likelihood, the state of our eliminatory systems is the most influential factor controlling the health of our assimilations. How does it work? We need to recognize that inadequate eliminations through any of the channels of elimination create an excess of toxins or poisons that should have been removed from the body. These toxins remain in the bloodstream or are deposited in the body tissues, not as food but as what Cayce called "drosses." The consciousness of the assimilatory organs is hampered by such drosses, and the process of regeneration fails, even if only to a minor degree—and this failure is the beginning of disease.

The benefits of proper elimination are well illustrated by the story of a sixty-three-year-old woman patient of mine who complained of tiredness. When I examined her, I found that she was anemic, with a hemoglobin count of 9.5 grams. So I started her on iron medication and kept her on it until two months later, when she developed a rash that I thought was due to the iron. Her hemoglobin was still only 9.5 grams, but I stopped the iron anyway. With an eye toward cleaning out the toxins that caused her rash, I suggested that she take an ounce of castor oil by mouth as a cathartic, then repeat the procedure in four days. Then I told her that I wanted to see her in a week.

My patient only partially heard my instructions. She took the castor oil at once, then repeated it in four days, and repeated it, and repeated it—until six weeks later, when she came in to see me. She still hadn't stopped taking the castor oil. It made her feel so good, she said. Her rash was gone and she really felt great, and she looked good, too. I tested her hemoglobin, thinking I should start her back on iron. This time her hemoglobin was 13.4 grams! I forgot about the iron.

The problems of assimilation and elimination may be part of any number of disease syndromes, and, as might be expected, they were given a great deal of attention in the Cayce readings. The readings also stressed the benefits of exercise, massage, and manipulation on both assimilation and elimination. The relationship among these three key functions must be kept in mind, if we are to rebuild the body or to maintain a state of health.

The following chapter discusses exercise, manipulation, and massage.

Diet Suggestions

In one of his readings, Cayce gave the following diet as one of the major points of a therapy program that included osteopathic manipulations, enemas, and a variety of mild cathartics. It seems to me an excellent aid toward establishing a basic diet for almost anyone:

MORNINGS: Citrus fruit juices or dry cereals with milk, but do not eat the cereals and the citrus fruit juices at the same meals; else we will find we change the activity of citrus fruit juices with the gastric juices of the stomach, by combining those that are acid and those that are alkaline reacting but of an acid nature. Crisp bacon, brown toast of whole wheat. Graham crackers, coddled egg, stewed fruit, fresh fruit; all of these are well, but not all at one meal to be sure.

NOONS: Preferably a green and fresh green vegetable salad; as tomatoes, celery, lettuce, peppers, radishes, carrots and the like. These should be grated together or chopped very fine. An oil salad dressing may be used.

EVENINGS: A general vegetable diet, well-balanced with three vegetables above the ground to one grown below. Well-cooked and well-seasoned vegetables. And the meats should only include lamb, fowl or fish. Do not take shell fish, but the fresh water fish would be preferable to the salt fish, see? Mackerel, and the like, don't take; but the fresh water fish will be much better for the body. Some little condiments may be taken at this meal, if so desired. Be mindful that not too much sweets are taken, but sufficient that there may be created a balance with the green vegetables for a sufficient fermentation in the proper proportion and nature. Hence tarts or fruit pies, or rolls, or the like; but not just cake alone, for this is not so well. Coffee and tea in moderation.

549-1

At the A.R.E. Clinic we have designed a "Basic Diet" that we use extensively as the starting point for most individuals. It can be followed strictly as a weight-control diet that is safe and helpful; or it can be expanded to accomplish whatever the person in charge of primary care wishes to do with it.

Another interesting idea about diet from the Cayce readings is his suggestion that there is a need for the body to ingest food that holds some of the local minerals or vibrations of the place where one lives.

In discussing therapy for various diseases in his state of extended consciousness, Cayce usually followed a basic diet plan that included no white sugar or white flour, no fried foods, and no pork, and it was very restrictive on sweets. Recommended were lots of fresh fruits, vegetables, and salads, and fish, fowl, and lamb for protein. Important variations would be taken to make the diet tend toward either the alkaline or the acid-ash balance, depending on the needs of the individual. For conditions where the body was overacid in its tissues, Cayce suggested a

much more alkaline diet. Frequent causes for such
overacidity were emotional upset, inadequate sleep
or exercise, illness, or excessive intake of sweets and
starches.

Among the dietary instructions and recommendations in the Cayce readings were a wide variety of
special foods and herbs that were indicated for their
special qualities. Among these were Jerusalem arti-
chokes, grape juice, onions, gelatin, wild ginseng,
wild cherry bark, sarsaparilla root, black snake root,
syrup of rhubarb, and yellow saffron. These recommended foods and herbs serve to purify, rebuild,
revitalize, and heal the body.

Vitamins

Vitamins were not neglected or downgraded in the
Cayce material; but the readings do suggest that it
is best to get one's vitamins from food if possible. It
is important to remember that food in the early
years of this century was far richer in vitamins, and
far poorer in the additives and chemicals that plague
our food today. The following extract from the Cayce
readings, while quite long, does give an interesting
picture of what he had to say about vitamins:

Q-12: What relation do the vitamins bear to the
glands? Give specific vitamins affecting
specific glands.

A-12: You want a book written on these!

They are food for same. Vitamins are that
from which the glands take those necessary influences to supply the energies to
enable the varied organs of the body to
reproduce themselves. Would it ever be considered that your toenails would be repro-
duced by the same as would supply the
breast, the head or the face? or that the
cuticle would be supplied from the same
as would supply the organ of the heart
itself? These are taken from GLANDS that
control the assimilated foods, and hence

A-12: the necessary elements or vitamins in same
to supply the various forces for enabling
each organ, each functioning of the body
to carry on in its creative or generative
forces, see?

These will begin with A—that supplies portions to the nerves, to bone, to the brain
force itself; not all of this, but this is a
part of A.

B and B-1 supply the ability of the energies,
or the moving forces of the nerve and of
the white blood supply, as well as the white
nerve energy in the nerve force itself, the
brain itself, and the ability of the sympathetic or involuntary reflexes through the
body. Now this includes all, whether you
are wiggling your toes or your ears or batting your eye, or what! In these we have
that supplying to the chyle that ability for
it to control the influence of fats, which is
necessary (and this body has never had
enough of it!), to carry on the reproducing
of oils that prevent the tenseness of the
joints, or that prevent the joints from becoming atrophied or dry, or to creak. At
times the body has had some creaks!

In C we find that which supplies the necessary influences to the flexes of every nature,
or a heart reaction, or a kidney contraction,
or the liver contraction, or the opening or
shutting of your mouth, the batting of the
eye, or the supplying of the saliva and the
muscular forces in face. These are all supplied by C,—not that it is the only supply,
but a part of same. It is that from which
the structural portions of the body are
stored, and drawn upon when it becomes
necessary. And when it becomes detrimental, or there is a deficiency of same—which
has been for this body—it is necessary to
supply same in such proportions as to aid;

A-12:   else the conditions become such that there
        are the bad eliminations from the incoordi-
        nation of the excretory functioning of the
        alimentary canal, as well as the heart, liver
        and lungs, through the expelling of those
        forces that are a part of the structural por-
        tion of the body.

        G supplies the general energies, or the sym-
        pathetic forces of the body itself.*

        These are the principles.

                                              2072–9

Fasting

Fasting involves complete abstinence from food,
or the use of diets wherein partial exclusion of food
substances is practiced. Throughout the ages, fasting
has been seen as a means of spiritual growth in the
practices of many religions; as a protest against civil
injustices or the alleged injustice of the law of the
land; as a means of binding an oath to seek revenge
or to defend one's honor; and, in more recent years,
as a means of preparation for a surgical procedure.

In the context of the Cayce readings, however,
fasting becomes something quite different. It becomes a setting aside of our own concepts of what or
how something should be done. It serves as an opportunity for an individual to allow himself to become *a channel through which God may work.* It
is a supplying of energy to the body that promotes
the coordination of organs and systems and enhances
assimilation and elimination. Thus, in purifying a
mind that is in a condition of mental confusion,

Vitamin G/Riboflavin. The heat-stable factor of the vitamin B complex. It functions as a coenzyme, or an active
prosthetic group of flavoproteins, concerned with oxida-
tive processes. It occurs in milk, muscle, liver, kidney,
eggs, grass, and various algae.
    Riboflavin promotes the growth of rats and prevents the
occurrence of a nutritional cataract in rats and a specific
dermatitis in turkeys; it is an essential nutrient for man,
the requirement being related to body size, metabolic rate,
and growth rate.

fasting accompanied by prayer is a mechanism of the mind, not of the body or of the diet. It is man bringing himself to low estate, abasing himself in order that the creative force of God might be made manifest.

What about Proof?

Not too long ago, an A.R.E. member from Minneapolis reported on her use of the herb mullein. She grows her own mullein in her backyard garden, spotted here and there among the lettuce and carrots. When her husband developed what was called a thrombophlebitis of the right ankle, their doctor prescribed some medication. However, both the patient and his wife wanted to use the remedy of mullein tea that Edgar Cayce had suggested so frequently in his readings. The patient's response to the tea was excellent, so he never took more than the first doses of the medicine that had been prescribed.

The question might rightly be asked: Why hasn't mullein been researched? The answer depends upon the definition of *research* that one uses. Mullein has been used for thousands of years—as have a multitude of other herbs. In the past, doctors and patients observed what happened when a person who was ill used the herb. They saw that the herb either worked or it didn't. This is what today we would call clinical observation. But today is also the day of "double-blind" statistical studies, and a therapy has little chance of survival unless it can wend its way through the double-blind.

"What is proof?" Einstein himself declined to answer that question; and Max Planck, the noted physicist, stated:

. . . new scientific truth does not triumph by convincing its opponents and making them see the light; but rather, because its opponents eventually die and a new generation grows up that is familiar with it.

And so it is with much of the Cayce suggestions on diet and nutrition.

Chapter Eleven
EXERCISE, MANIPULATION AND MASSAGE

The life force residing within each of us must manifest itself through action in this world. Action means movement, and it is only through movement and flexibility that the energy of life is kept flowing freely through our bodies. Movement of the body comes about through our daily activities, but it is the stretching, the reaching of limits of motion, that can come only through actions that we would classify as exercise or through some form of manipulation or massage, that brings to us our greatest benefit.

Man's activity on Earth is expressed through his conscious muscular movements, whether they direct his voice, his hands or feet, or whatever. Indeed, if he had no ability to control these muscles, which we call striated muscles, he could not influence the world around him. Perhaps he could use his mind as a tool, and send out thought waves, but he could not direct his physical body. The body-in-action is an overt manifestation of the individual life in this world and in this dimension.

When the human body is quiet—when it is asleep— the outside, muscular activities are essentially absent. However, life is still present, and activities are directed inward instead of outward. Digestion is progressing, food is being converted into energy to build up the body, the organs of elimination are acting on wastes to be gotten rid of, the heart and the lungs continue their incessant jobs, and the nervous system is busy conducting these affairs as well as dreaming up a storm and helping the individual to gain guidance and direction in his life.

The Cayce readings emphasize the importance of

both the autonomic nervous system, which moves
and regulates the internally functioning organs and
systems, and the cerebrospinal nervous system, which
moves and regulates our external muscular movements. The autonomic is the mediator and director
of the life force within the human body, an unconscious system that gives us the ability to *have* life in
this dimension. The cerebrospinal, on the other hand,
gives us the ability to consciously *manifest* that life
in constructive—or destructive—activities in the world
around us. Both are necessary, and both fulfill their
destiny in the normal, active human being.

Cayce often suggested that when a person's autonomic system was not coordinated with the cerebrospinal system—or when it was disturbed within
itself—trouble resulted. This trouble he called disease, which, if persisted in, then became a disease
or a structural illness. It was the need within the
body for a coordinated relationship between these
two portions of the nervous system that brought
about repeated recommendations in the readings
for activities that would restore such coordination
and help to bring about a healing. The need for
coordination exists not only between the nervous
systems but among the various functioning organs
as well as within the real structure of the human
being:

> And as is then to be understood, these MUST
> coordinate and cooperate—body, mind, soul—if
> there is to be the best reaction in the physical,
> mental or spiritual.
>
> 1189-2

It is important to recognize that exercise, massage,
and manipulation are related. Each is active in moving the structural parts of the body in its own specific way. They all influence the relative integrity of
the activity within the nervous systems of the body;
they all have an influence on the activity of the
lymphatics as well as the eliminations of the body
associated with the lymph; and they all aid in bringing about a coordination among various activities

within the body. Each has its place in the healing process. Exercise, of course, is what one can do at any time without assistance. Massage and manipulation, however, require the aid of a therapist, an expert in the art. But all are beneficial, all are helpful, and all can play a critical role in the healing of the body and the maintenance of its well-being.

Exercise

The consciousness of the American people over the past two decades has sent multitudes of joggers out into the early morning or late evening hours to jog and jog and jog. And the health of the American people has increased—heart conditions have improved, weight has dropped, and the general state of well-being has taken a sharp upward turn. The more conservative of these health seekers have walked instead of jogged or run, and they likewise have seen the positive results of their efforts.

In the Cayce readings, walking was the most commonly suggested single exercise: 163 readings were given recommending walking as part of a therapy program for everything from arthritis and circulatory problems to neuritis, incoordination, obesity, and toxemia. In seventeen instances, walking was suggested to women who were pregnant, and frequently came the injunction that "walking is the best exercise" (2582–4), or "the exercise of walking is the best." (2759–1) To a young man who did not sleep well, was anemic, and tended to have symptoms of arthritis, Cayce responded:

Q-7: What exercise should the body take in order to increase the weight and help lungs?

A-7: First purify the system and let the exercises come along afterwards; not while the body is being adjusted from the conditions existent in the present.

Walking, of course; and working, is the best exercise.

Q-8:   Recommend some sport.

A-8:   Running, walking, golfing, fishing or the like.

                                                              2157-2

For an underweight, asthenic young woman of twenty, Cayce suggested "1–2 hours alone in a walk in the open daily with mental forces directed to building physically." 136–3

Don't exercise so as to cause stress or irritation to the body—that seems reasonable, but it is very important to remember. Don't overtax the body. But how much walking is important for the average person? With a bit of frustration, perhaps, at his suggestions not being taken, Cayce said to one man: "Whether it's a mile or a step, do that which makes for a better 'feel' for the body; getting into the open." (257–204) It was further understood—and stated—in the readings that the walking should not be done too soon after eating, if the body is to be exercised to the extent that it becomes overheated.

It is generally accepted today that walking can be taken as an exercise and thus can be done more vigorously than leisurely. A good rule is to walk to increase the pulse rate to the proper level for you. How is this determined? Subtract your age from the number 220, then take 70–85% of the result: your pulse rate should be within the resulting range for optimum effect on your vascular system and your body. For instance, if you are 55 years old, subtract 55 from 220, leaving 165; 70% of that is 116; 85% of 165 is 140. You should walk, then, rapidly enough to increase your pulse rate to somewhere between 116 and 140. If you are not well, then you should proceed very slowly until you can work up to that level.

How long should you walk? Perhaps half an hour a day at least three times a week. Take your pulse at the carotid artery in the neck—that's the easiest place. And, if you'd like to find a pace you could use to get started on this activity, use your watch and take 55 to 65 left-foot paces a minute. (The right

foot normally follows!) Observe how good you feel
when you're done. According to the readings, walking should be done vigorously and long enough—
about half an hour—to bring about a sweat on the
body.

Cayce told a thirty-seven-year-old man whose blood
sugar was a bit high that the best exercise for him
would be "a walking exercise, and the general set-
ting-up exercise—that above the waist for mornings
(arms, etc.), and that below the waist for evenings,
these are preferable ones for the body." (2772-3)
Other exercises, of course, are beneficial: jogging,
running, tennis, swimming, and many others. An
arthritic man, just thirty-one years old, was told to
"get in the water, though, as soon as possible; for
the ability to make movements in the water will be
beneficial to the internal circulatory forces. (849-32)

In my own work with many individuals who would
like to expand their useful and vital years, I have
encouraged them to do exercises that will keep the
spine flexible. Cayce suggested that the one movement that will make for longevity better than any
other is the stretching movement of the cat.

Dr. Rex Conyers, director of the Osteopathic Research Division of the Edgar Cayce Foundation, advised those adopting an exercise program to begin
with this affirmation: "Father, God, I will that this
activity create in me a greater channel that thy will
be done." Listed below are three exercises suggested
by Dr. Conyers that give you an indication of what
he thinks would be beneficial for every person:

Vertical: Stand with feet apart. Stretch on your
toes and while doing so breathe deeply. Stretch
your arms one at a time as high as you can, and
while stretching make a fist. Stretch them alternating in this manner while coming up on your
toes and breathing deeply.

Vertical: Place your forearms on your hips, rise
up on your toes, and then do deep knee bends to
the count of three. After a short period of time,
you will be able to maintain your balance quite

easily. You should inhalf deeply as you rise on your toes and then exhale completely as you do the complete "squat." Then inhale deeply as you come to the upright position again, attempting to stay on your toes. Exhale once again as you bend your knees to the squatting position. Repeat this exercise as often as you wish.

Sitting: Begin by sitting on the floor with legs outstretched in front of you as far as possible. First, bend forward from the waist and reach for one outstretched foot with both hands. Hold the tension for a few seconds, then release and sit back, with hands in your lap or at your sides. Then repeat the stretching movement, grasping for the other foot, holding the tension, and return to sitting position with body erect. Repeat this exercise several times.

Conyers points out that the readings imply rather strongly that the vertical exercises should be done in the morning upon arising from sleep, while the horizontal exercises should be done in the evening before retiring.

It seems that certain inhabitants of the jungle naturally perform exercises that keep them healthy and strong—at least in part. Have you ever seen a member of the cat family s...t...r...e...t...c...h? I've watched the lion and the leopard in the Phoenix Zoo, as well as the cats that have at one time or another inhabited our home. They all awaken, lazily look around, yawn sometimes, then get up and stretch their muscles. The readings agree that this is good not only for cats but for most human beings.

Several exercises are part of the daily routine, and I teach these to my patients, for I know that many of them are faced with problems of limited time and all those tensions and pressures of present-day life. These exercises are aimed at creating a flexibility of the spine as well as a stretching and relaxation of the muscles along the spine and in the extremities. When the spine stays mobile and free of those limitations imposed by the vicissitudes of life, it stands to reason that nerve impulses to and from the cerebral cortex, to and from the autonomic nervous system (the unconscious mind), and to and from the general muscular and organic structures of the body will be more intelligible and more accurate in the instructions they carry to the receiving organs, than they would be if such exercises were never performed. Indeed, the body tends to crystallize when inactive: for example, an elbow will become permanently bent and, to an extent, unusable if left with the elbow flexed in a cast too long.

A Morning Exercise Program

First: Stretching like a cat comes most easily just after getting out of bed. Exercising like a cat, according to Cayce, lengthens one's life. Therefore, one might assume Cayce was implying that the stretching exercise, consistently utilized, produces a continued upgrading of the total health of the body.

Second: The head and neck exercise tones up the sensorium of the body. We perceive this Earth dimension only through our senses; and, if we have a purpose here that is significant, we had best stay in touch with this world and its activities as they surround and impact us. Sight, hearing, taste, touch, and smell—all these are apparently toned up and made better by using this exercise.

Cayce always suggested that we use any kind of repetitive therapy with patience, persistence, and consistency. Over a period of months and years, then, the effect on the senses will be seen, as will be a greater degree of balance between the cerebrospinal and the autonomic nervous systems, consequently improving their organic function—which in turn improves vitality and length of life.

A reading dealing with poor vision describes how Cayce would have you do this exercise and how it may be of benefit:

When we remove the pressures of the toxic forces we will improve the vision. Also the head and neck exercise will be most helpful. Take this regularly, not taking it sometimes and leaving off sometimes, but each morning and each evening take this exercise regularly for six months and we will see a great deal of difference. Sitting erect, bend the head forward three times, to the back three times, to the right side three times, to the left side three times, and then circle the head each way three times. Don't hurry through with it, but take the time to do it. We will get results.

3549–1

Third: In my morning preparation there is also a group of movements designed to keep the dorsal and lumbar spine flexible, much as the head and neck exercise keeps the cervical spine mobile. One may begin with any one of the three basic movements. I usually do each one about fifteen or twenty times, but that is a matter of personal choice.

One is an anterior-posterior exercise: standing upright, with feet fairly close together, one extends both hands overhead and reaches back as far as possible, bending backward. Then the movement is forward, reaching down and touching the toes without bending one's knees any more than necessary.

The second movement is a side-to-side exercise, not twisting, but bending laterally first to the right and then to the left, keeping the face straight forward, and reaching down alongside the body with the hand and arm as the body is bent in that direction.

This third movement has been called the "big swing." In doing this, one stands with feet about twelve to fifteen inches apart, stretching the arms straight out to the sides. Then the body is twisted first to the right, following the swing with the head and eyes as much as possible, and letting the arms swing laterally rather vigorously, in a sense pulling the rest of the body in the twisting movement. When the full twisting motion stops, it is then reversed completely around to the left, and the big swing continues until the desired number of the double swings is completed.

Fourth: Here is an exercise borrowed from the Chinese. Its purpose is to promote better eyesight. I massage acupuncture points around the eye seven times in one circular direction, then seven times in the opposite direction. The massage above the eyebrow is simply in one direction laterally from the center point. There is no circular direction there.

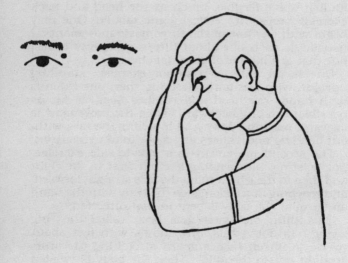

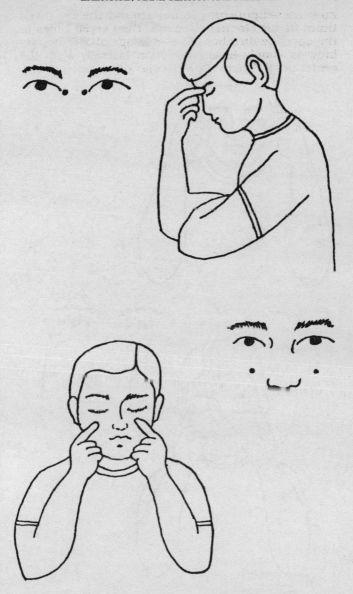

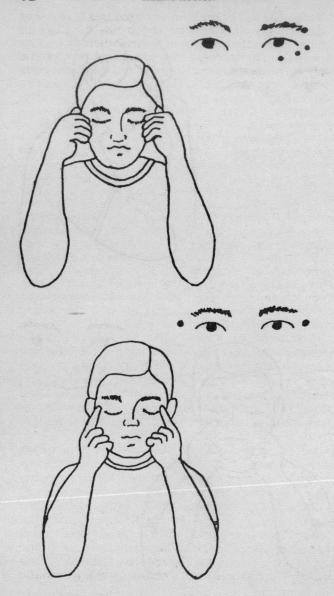

Fifth: The last of my morning exercises is one that I devised myself. However, it too has its roots in China, where the concept of auriculotherapy had its inception. This therapy can affect any part of the body through the use of needles or transcutaneous electrotherapy applied to the human ear. The entire body is represented on the ear, and there are doctors who limit their entire therapy program to treatment of the ear.

The exercise is performed by grasping both ears—right ear with right hand, left ear with left hand—so that the palm is flat against the entire ear and the fingers hold the earlobe firmly against the palm of the hand. Then both ears are rotated at the same time in a circular fashion, moving them in this manner as firmly as one finds reasonably comfortable. One should not hurt the ear, but movement is essential. The ears may be rotated in this manner twenty-five to fifty times in one direction, then the same number of times in the opposite direction. Then, without removing the hands, and with the elbows akimbo, pressure should be applied against the ear from both sides simultaneously, the same number of times.

The circular movement of the ear acts as a gentle balancing stimulation to all the auriculotherapy points of the ear, giving the body, in a very real sense, an over-all toning up. The last pressure exercise tends to increase the pressure in the internal canal of the ear, thus producing a gentle exercise on the eardrum itself and a stimulation of the lining of the internal canal.

Exercise is important to the body, and that which comes about in one's daily work is seldom sufficient to keep the spine mobile and the neurological impulses flowing without obstruction or hindrance. Sufficient exercise, done on a regular, scheduled basis, can largely eliminate the need for manipulations or massages, for all three really are effective on the same basis—that is, influencing the muscle tone and vitality, stretching the tendons and mobilizing the bony structures, and enhancing the lymphatic flow and the neurological impulses and communication.

When you start exercising, however, make it the kind of exercise that you will continue, preferably, for the rest of your life. For if you begin an exercise and then stop, your body will rebel, which is just what the exercise is designed to eliminate—rebellions of the very consciousness of the tissues of the human body.

Manipulation

Manipulation may be viewed through the Cayce material as part of the armamentarium for bringing the body back to a balance. Differing from exercise, it is administered by another party—not by the one who would receive the benefit. Differing also from massage, manipulation is more definite, oriented more to specific passive joint movement and to rearrangement, in a sense, of large muscle masses.

Cayce did not always recommend manipulations to start with—instead, at times he suggested, in the case of a toxic or weak person, a course of eliminations or strengthening before this kind of therapy was begun. And, of course, there were thousands of instances where manipulations were not even mentioned. There are conditions of the body, however, that will not ordinarily be corrected without manipulative or adjustment therapy, and Cayce was very firm on that point.

From the readings, it appears that the osteopathy of his day was superior to other methods of corrective manipulation. Today, however, not only are some medical doctors turning serious attention to such manipulative techniques, but some osteopaths, chiropractors, and medical doctors are doing cranial therapy; and a variety of differing mechanical corrective techniques are crossing over previous medical, professional barriers. So, it might be said that when someone has a problem that may respond to manipulations or adjustments, it would be well to recognize the abilities of the therapist as being more

important than the particular method he uses or
the professional degree he carries.

The picture that emerges from the Cayce material,
however, is one where osteopathy creates a balance
in the body, a coordination, a release of energy in
the tissues at times, but holding back the energies
where it is proper to do so. Osteopathic treatments
stimulate the fluids, the organs, the cells—even the
atoms—of the body, to function correctly, in coordination with other parts of the system, in a balance,
a harmony of action, of life itself.

In maintaining a balanced viewpoint, we should
remember that these treatments—like some medicines, like castor oil packs, like massage or exercise,
like visual imagery or prayer—are only corrective or
stimulatory and are not really healing in nature.
Cayce pointed this out to one person:

> Remember, mechanical [osteopathic] adjustments,
> like even properties as may be taken of the medici-
> nal nature, are only correctives—and NATURE or
> the DIVINE force, does the healing.
>
> 1467–9

In the readings, osteopathy covered a wide scope
of value in treatment. Serious conditions, such as
seizure problems (epilepsy), were specifically steered
toward manipulative treatments; but this kind of
therapy was suggested also as a health-maintenance
procedure. The osteopathic lesion—sometimes thought
of as a patch of nerve cells in a sac of lymphatic
fluid—was often said to have played a specific part
in a variety of illnesses. Cayce saw instances of epilepsy that he said were caused by such lesions and
that could be cleared up by osteopathic treatments,
diet, and castor oil packs placed over the abdomen.
These instances of seizure activity had their etiology,
or cause, in osteopathic lesions in the abdomen or
alongside the spine—not, as generally thought, in
the brain. The rationale for such treatments involved
release of pressures alongside the spine where the
spinal nerves exit from the spinal cord; the alter-
ation of the body acid-base balance through dietary

regimens; and the improvement of lymphatic flow and utilization of foods in the abdominal cavity through the use of castor oil packs.

Such therapeutic programs often fail because the individuals and those aiding the patients do not proceed with the patience, persistence, and consistency that is required. For it takes time and molecular-cellular change in order to restore normalcy from a cellular abnormality. It is a good example of how Cayce's suggestions follow a course of regeneration in the physiology of the body, rather than a scarring or an overlying medication. It is a restoration of normal—but the results are not easily obtained when the illness is deeply set. Yet, it is possible.

Cayce's balanced point of view probably can best be illustrated by the following comment:

> As we would find, it would be advisable to continue the osteopathic treatments at least twice each week; for, while healing of any nature must be from within, it depends upon the attitude taken toward all elements and influences within the experience as to a manifestation of life in the material plane. In the physical body, as we have given, each atom is a whole universe in itself, and is a portion of the whole. When there is coordination within self, in the *inner* self—when the inner shrine receives the impulse, then healing is complete; yet each atomic influence receives an impulse from various forms of application to a material body, or to a material demonstration or manifestation of a spiritual influence animating *through* a material body.
>
> 275–32

MASSAGE

In the Cayce readings, massage was suggested more frequently than any other form of therapy. Dr. Harold Reilly, a therapist to whom Cayce sent hundreds of people, is credited with the statement that "one massage is equivalent to a four-mile walk." It depends, of course, on the type of massage, and I'm sure Dr.

Reilly was talking about the increased circulation that comes about as a result of a massage and the improved neurological communication, for a massage sends literally millions of impulses throughout the neurological pathways of the body.

Cayce not only suggested full-body massages but frequently gave information about localized massages that have benefit. The following extract from the readings points toward the feet as beneficiaries in this instance and what might happen as a result:

> The massages as we find are very, very good. We would massage more in the bursa of the feet; as under the toe, in the instep and in the heel. The increasing of stimulation in this direction will cause the nerves of the ends of the sciatics to be enlivened. This will make twitching sensations at times in the calf of the leg, under the knees, and in the thighs, but these will not be too aggravating—and will indicate to the body that there is being reestablished the communication, as it might be called, between the lower limbs or the locomotories and body-forces.
>
> 2778–6

Massage is an important therapy in our program at the A.R.E. Clinic, and, in the context of the Edgar Cayce readings, it has been recommended for a variety of problems.

Tension, stress, and lifestyle pressures produce for many human bodies a condition that I would call a problem of assimilation. This may or may not be associated with an ulcer of the stomach, but often it is diagnosed as hyperacidity. And the problem really is one of inability—because of those stresses— to take food into the digestive tract and change it adequately so that it can be absorbed into the cells of the intestinal wall and thus into the bloodstream or lymphatics; again changed or made available to the cells of the body through the activity of the liver or the lymphatic centers through which it passes; and then passed on to the body proper, by means of the circulatory system, where it might be

utilized in repairing, recharging, rehabilitating, or
rebuilding the structure of the body. The inability
may lie in any one of a variety of stations where
these activities occur. If there is a lack of proper
function in any location, there is then a problem of
assimilation, with consequent lack of proper structure and thus of proper function in the human body.
It may be quite minimal, but nevertheless it is
present.

Without going into the details of how stress might
cause this type of syndrome, let us assume that it
has actually happened and see what Cayce might
say about it. I find two extracts particularly interesting, one of which deals with an area that is
important in the acupuncture arena—known as the
"Door of Life." It lies across the back, just below the
rib cage. You will find reference to it here, and the
suggestions have to do with mechanical-vibrator
massage, a device that can be obtained from any of
the large department stores or health food stores.

> These as we find were produced, and the condi-
> tions gradually built up, by the lack of the proper
> assimilation in the digestive forces of the body.

> If there would be the return to the diets, in rather
> a consistent manner as has been indicated, with
> the rubs occasionally for the circulation—you see—
> throughout, we would find much better condition
> for the body.

> We would find the condition would be very much
> improved by the use of the electrically driven vi-
> brator also, over the whole of the cerebrospinal
> system; extending especially to the lower limbs
> and making rather specific applications across
> the lumbar, the 9th dorsal and through the head
> and neck.

> 389—9

Then, to another person, this time in the first
reading given him, where problems existed in the
physical body, arising "from the great emotional
strains":

Each evening when ready to retire, apply for twenty minutes the electrically driven vibrator. Use the cup applicator down either side of the spine, as well as on the spine itself, from base of brain to the end of spine. After applying this thoroughly to spine, extend it across the area of the diaphragm from the back, you see—that is, crosswise the body on the lower portion of the rib area from the back. Then apply it across the sacral area, which is the lower portion of the back from the hip area, you see; and then apply it down the sciatic nerve along the thigh, and especially under knees and to the feet themselves. Take the time, not merely as something to be gotten through with.

2452-1

Massage is most commonly done with oil. Peanut oil was most frequently suggested in the Cayce material, and it has come to be highly regarded by those who have used it for rheumatic joints and aching muscles. We have used peanut oil in our Clinic for massage thousands of times, and we find it to be consistently remarkable in what it can sometimes do in the alleviation of human ills.

I have wondered just what physiological mechanisms are involved in massage. How does it act in or on the human body? Does it produce those effects that Cayce describes as "vibratory"? In reviewing some Cayce material, I came across the following material that threw some light not only on my wonderings but on peanut oil:

The "why" of massage should be considered: Inactivity causes many of those portions along the spine from which impulses are received to the various organs to be lax, or taut, or allow some to receive greater impulses than others. The massage aids the ganglia to receive impulses from nerve forces as it aids circulation through the various portions of the organism.

2456-4

and also:

> Daily, for at least half to an hour and a half,
> massage the body; not rudely, not crudely, not
> with the attempt to make adjustment—for many
> weeks yet. Massage with Peanut oil,—yes, the
> lowly Peanut oil has in its combination that which
> will aid in creating in the superficial circulation,
> and in the superficial structural forces, as well as
> in the skin and blood, those influences that make
> more pliable the skin, muscles, nerves and ten-
> dons, that go to make up the assistance to struc-
> tural portions of the body. Its absorption and its
> radiation through the body will also strengthen
> the activities of the structural body itself.
>
> 2968—1

The Cayce readings dealt with specifics many times,
for many people, but apparently never gave a routine
that might be followed for the average person in
need of a general massage.Over the years, building
with our experience on the information Dr. Reilly
has developed, we have created procedures for doing
a full-body massage, for it became necessary for us
to teach family members in the art of massage so
that they could continue a treatment regimen at
home, having once started it in the Clinic.

The A-B-C's of Massage

EQUIPMENT NEEDED:
1. Table—30 inches wide, and firm, at convenient height.
2. Two sheets and two pillows (one pillow for
   head and the other under knees).
3. Oil. Made up as follows:
   1 teaspoon lanolin dissolved in
   6 ounces peanut oil, add
   2 ounces olive oil and
   2 ounces rose water.

GENERAL DIRECTIONS:
1. Wash hands.
2. Begin with a friendly touch.

3. Order of general massage: neck, arms, front of legs, abdomen, back of legs, back. This may be altered for particular reasons.
4. Maintain constant touch with subject.
5. Be alert to pain, tenderness, or stiffness, and massage accordingly.
6. Encourage relaxation on the part of the subject and do not encourage talking. If the subject wants to talk some, it is all right. But do not get into controversial subjects or introduce new subjects. If patient is stimulated from talking, he loses some of the benefit of massage.
7. Do not hurt the patient. Watch the face for signals of pain or discomfort.
8. Use both hands rhythmically, keeping the fingers together and shaping them around the body. Do not "dig in."
9. Make firm strokes toward the heart and light strokes away from the heart.
10. Use "Tender Loving Care."
11. General massage is geared to 40 or 45 minutes.

MASSAGE METHODS:
1. With long strokes, apply enough oil so that the hands move smoothly on patient's skin.
2. NECK:
   To protect a woman's hair from the oil, it is good to wrap the hair up in a towel that can be fastened with Scotch tape or a large safety pin. Work standing at the head of the subject. Cradle the head in one hand and massage along the lymph channels of the neck under the ear going toward the chest and shoulder. Turn the head the other way and do the opposite side. Place fingers under the neck at the base of the skull. The tips of the fingers are on each side of the vertebrae. Use "W" movements working from the base of the skull to as low under the shoulders as is comfortable. Work out to the shoulders and then come back to the base of the skull with a smooth

stroking motion. This can be done three times.
Finish up with several strokes moving slowly
down the neck and then back up with very
light pressure.

3. ARM:
    Upper Arm: Begin massaging around the
    shoulder, making firm strokes toward the
    heart, light strokes away from the heart. The
    strokes of the hands dovetail, gently moving
    and warming the flesh.
    Forearm: Bend at the elbow and continue
    dovetail strokes toward the heart.
    Hand: Stroke fingers toward the heart and
    stretch the palm of hand. Work each finger
    separately. Proceed with wrist, elbow, and
    shoulder joint movements. Make nerve pres-
    sures with thumbs and fingers from shoul-
    der to wrist, omitting the inside elbow area,
    counting 1-2 while doing each pressure. End
    arm massage with long, firm strokes from
    wrist to shoulder and return with a light,
    warm, slow stroke.

4. LEGS:
    Hip Joint: Work along the hip joint with deep
    circular strokes.
    Thighs: Work well along the side and top of
    the thigh. Use the deep stroking and knead-
    ing motion toward the heart that you used
    for the upper arm. For the inner thigh, use a
    wringing up-and-down movement as well. It
    is less tiring for masseuse or masseur to use
    a knee-and-body, back-and-forth movement
    while massaging.
    Knee Cap: Massage above the knee cap with
    the thumbs in a semicircular motion, around
    the sides with circular strokes.
    Lower Leg: Work on either side of the shin
    bone with a rolling, kneading stroke. Avoid
    pressure on bone.
    Feet: Work around the ankle bones with tips
    of fingers. Use palms of hands on bottoms of
    feet as if rolling a ball between the hands.
    Massage heels, sides, ball, and instep of feet.

Always work toward the heart. Each toe can be pulled and stretched gently. End massage of leg with long, firm strokes from ankle to hip, returning with a low, light stroke. For some subjects, a gentle pull and shake of the entire leg is beneficial.

5.   ABDOMEN:

Always use a clockwise motion on the abdomen. Use a large circular motion over colon areas with pressure always going clockwise. Vibrate colon with clockwise pressure.

Under each side of the rib cage, massage away from the heart with small semicircular strokes.

Work on each side of waist with an up-and-down motion. Avoid hip bone. Vibrate liver and pancreas areas by placing hands under and over rib cage.

Stroke off with a movement from the back upward toward the abdomen at the waist. Then have the patient turn over onto his tummy.

6.   BACKS OF LEGS:

Thigh: Remembering to keep the pressure strokes upward toward the heart, massage the thigh beginning on the outside near the buttocks. With rhythmic strokes by both hand, one after the other, work down the thigh. The inside of the thigh should be kneaded with an up-and-down wringing, rolling stroke.

Back of Knee: Drain the back of the knee with upward strokes in X-like motion.

Lower Leg: After massaging the calf of the leg (with dovetail strokes), the leg should then be bent at the knee and massaged. Thus, gravity aids the draining of the leg. Work the ankle joint around and up and down. Begin nerve pressures on the back of the leg, starting under the buttocks and moving toward the ankle, omitting the area behind the knee. Finally, use long strokes up to the buttocks and soft stroking movements down to the ankle to stroke off and finish.

7. BACK:
    Divide the back into two sections: the upper
    back (cervical area to ninth dorsal, which is
    found an inch below the base of the scapula)
    and the lower back (sacrum to ninth dorsal).
    Upper Back: Draw hearts with the flats of
    the fingers, right hand on right side of spine,
    left hand on left side of spine, starting at the
    neck and going down to the ninth dorsal.
    Sometimes on a heavy or muscular person,
    or where special attention is needed, it is
    better to work one side at a time. Do the
    same area at least three times, then make
    the strokes larger until the whole width of
    the back is stretched.
    Lower Back: Massage the lower back in the
    same way, using heart-shaped strokes, but
    work from the sacrum *up* to the ninth dorsal.
    Sides and Shoulders of Back: Work on
    the sides of the body, making up-and-down
    strokes moving up the sides toward the arm-
    pits, and large circular motions around the
    shoulders and shoulder blades and down along
    the muscular areas to the buttocks. Do this
    on both sides, working across the body for
    one side and then moving around to the other
    side of the table for the second side.
    Buttocks: Massage the buttocks and aim for
    stimulation of the sciatic nerve deep in the
    tissues.
    Completing Manipulation of Back: Press on
    each side of vertebrae moving from base of
    skull to ninth dorsal and from the sacrum
    back to the ninth dorsal. When congestion is
    felt, press for 12 seconds. A continuous move-
    ment in these areas milks the lymphatics of
    the spinal column.
       Then stand at the head of the subject. Plac-
    ing both hands, one on each side of the spine
    just below the neck, lean on the palms and
    move them slowly down the back and past
    the sacrum before coming back up the back

with a light stroking on either side. Do this three times, the last time with very light pressure.

Remember to keep contact with the subject and that relaxation, lymphatic cleansing, and balancing of the nervous systems are the aims of massage!

Chapter Twelve
PRAYER AND MEDITATION

Healing of the human body might best be called a growth in consciousness, a new awareness of the Divine within one's being. True healing, according to the Cayce readings, is always an adventure in consciousness leading to new understandings. Cayce suggested that a healing of the physical body that does not provide one with hope in the spiritual nature of his being is "saving a body for destruction in materiality." The two most common and widely used adventures that join the material to the spiritual are prayer and meditation. Both prayer and meditation are recommended and used regularly by most of the patients who come to the A.R.E. Clinic for upgrading of their physical bodies.

From the readings came information that would lead one to think that any person, really, who sincerely desires to bring to someone else that growth of consciousness that characterizes all true healing is undoubtedly among those who have been called to the priesthood of healing. Whether he or she has a medical degree is of little importance. Of utmost significance, however, is that the fruits of the spirit must become part of the healer's total activities.

Prayer

The cultivation of spiritual insights is the activity that goes on unconsciously as one prays or as one meditates. Prayer need not be of the silent or of the verbal type. It may be an action, such as the laying on of hands, the process that passes energy on to another individual, which brings about some degree of healing. Dr. Arthur Bernstein, president of the Essex County, New Jersey, Medical Society, has several ideas on this subject.

He draws from an article in the *British Medical Journal* that describes the no-touching problem in England—a problem that is undoubtedly prevalent in all Anglo-Saxon countries. "We have lost the ability to comfort one another, and we have a cold attitude towards strangers and foreigners. . . . This brings about frequent need for coming to the doctor's office to be examined." Bernstein apparently believes that this comes about as a result of people's fear of touching one another. He urges the physician to use more and more of the "laying on of hands" as a means of treating this kind of fear, this feeling of loneliness and estrangement.

Bernstein lifts the banner of his profession considerably higher as he states:

> The physician is not truly a "doctor" unless he can understand and forgive people their weaknesses. He must have the humility to recognize that we really know very little about human physiology and even less about human pharmacology. The physician must be patient with each of his patients. Whether they be moral or immoral according to his own concepts is not his problem. His function is to treat everyone with respect in order to re-establish the human dignity of the patient in his dark hours.

In the Edgar Cayce readings, there has been much given about forgiveness, which Bernstein believes must be part of the "true doctor's" makeup. The following extract from one of the readings speaks pertinently to this concept:

> To be sure, others have apparently had ideals and have fallen far short of living up to such ideals. . . .

Yet ye know in whom and in what ye have believed.
And as He was and is willing to forgive, so much
the entity within self be willing and capable and
desirous of forgiving—even as the entity would be
forgiven. . . .

Then to not forgive would be giving way to self in
such a manner as to become even worse than
those that in the moment of self-delusionment
gave way in those ways that brought—or bring—
this disturbance or unsettlement in the experience of this body.

As ye would that others would forgive you, even so
must you forgive—if you would find peace, that
harmony within self. And thus may ye help those;
not condoning, no—but not condemning either.
For, to condemn is to become as a party to such.
And with that measure ye condemn others, ye are
guilty of that condemnation.

                                        2293–3

Bernstein perhaps is not aware of the energies
that may pass from one individual to another that
bring healing to the human body, but he *is* aware of
understanding, compassion, tenderness, love, patience, and forgiveness—all of which are portions of
that which the Bible loosely gathers under the title
of the fruits of the Spirit or Love itself. And that
Love is the greatest healing force of the human spirit
and the physical body.

Prayer and healing have been evidenced throughout the centuries as having a cause-and-effect relationship, but to prove it is another matter. It is a
difficult thing to consider how one might translate
Divine action into "acceptable" scientific data. Prayer
has been called "talking to God," but it is certainly
more than that. We don't really know all that a prayer
might be, and we are hard put to understand the
nature of Divine action in the healing process.

A doctor by the name of Playton Collipp recently
published a study on the efficacy of prayer in a
controlled study of young people who had leukemia.
He found that of ten youngsters who received prayers,

seven were still alive after fifteen months. Of the eight who were not prayed for, only two were alive after fifteen months. However, his study was subsequently criticized because the members of each group were not matched by age, by method of drug treatment, and by the type of leukemia.

Collipp responded that he was aware of these limitations before he wrote up his findings, but he stated, "I don't think they change the conclusions in the article at all." Collipp went on to say: "My final opinion is that the study supports the view that prayers are efficacious. It doesn't establish it, but supports it. I think more studies ought to be done. I don't think God would mind."

The A.R.E. Clinic has an active program in healing prayer. Study groups in the Phoenix area are given monthly a list of the names of those who have asked to be healed. The list is reworked each month. One woman who has been in the A.R.E. for many years, and who is a patient at the Clinic, recently asked to be put on the prayer list. She had been in an accident nearly a year ago and barely managed to come out of it alive. Her recovery over the months, however, has been very encouraging. But she had a problem with her vision, which had never cleared up, and she did not know beforehand that the healing list existed. So she asked. Her problem was that she saw double all the time, one visual image being higher than the other unless she cocked her head to one side. She could not read, sew, or drive. It was not only exasperating, it was limiting her entire life effort. One week after her name was placed on the list, she came into the Clinic, reporting to her doctor that suddenly one morning her vision was normal when she awakened and has been good ever since.

One other story of healing comes from a very active A.R.E. member in middle America. In their prayer and healing group, they have used recently the laying on of hands when asked to do so and have had some definite reports of success. One woman had been told after an examination by her doctor that she had a probable cancer of the breast and that a biopsy

should be done. My correspondent was asked to be
the one to "channel" the healing energy from the
group to the subject.

> I felt the creative energies passing through (had
> placed my right hand on her forehead and the left
> hand on the neck at approximately the thyroid
> gland). There was much heat, not only in the
> hands but throughout the whole body. She felt
> the energies enter and felt the heat. Each member
> of the group said they felt the flow of energy . . .
> when she went for another examination at the
> hospital on Monday (the next day), she was exam-
> ined by four doctors. The lump had decreased in
> size to about the size of a very small pea, and it
> was decided that there was no reason to perform
> the biopsy at all. They were somewhat puzzled
> and asked what had happened. She told them
> about the laying on of hands. You can imagine
> the consternation. One, a woman doctor, followed
> our friend out of the examination room of the
> hospital and said that she had always been able
> to "see" a patient's illness before there was a physi-
> cal examination but had never told anyone be-
> cause she thought they'd think she had flipped
> her lid.

It's too bad that such occurrences are not more
widely accepted, but, on the other hand, it is good
that they are being reported and that more doctors
are becoming aware of their reality.

Meditation

Meditation is considered part of a healing process
because it is understood to be effective in bringing
the conscious part of oneself into a close attune-
ment with the Divine within, the God within one's
own being. Meditation is listening to the Divine in
the same sense that prayer is speaking to the Divine.
In meditation, the body becomes quiet and the mind
is gradually stilled. There is a movement of spiritual
energy upward from the base of the spine, touching

all seven of the spiritual centers that in Eastern
tradition have been called "chakras," and producing
a cleansing and balancing of those centers—and a
balancing of the entire body to the extent that the
meditation is effective. (See opposite page.)

Meditation is a discipline practiced by millions of
individuals throughout the world, producing, as
would be expected, a multitude of methods or procedures. All seem to have one thing in common,
however, in that they claim to attune one to that
part of oneself that lies within and that is considered to be holy, unspeakable, and Divine in its nature.

The level of consciousness that is tapped in states
of meditation has been called the "alpha" state. Lind-
say Jacob, a psychiatrist from Pittsburgh, discussed
relaxation at a 1973 medical symposium in Phoenix,
reporting on how one reaches the alpha state by the
process of relaxation described originally by Schultz
in his tome on autogenic training. The steps enumerated by Jacob prepare one for autogenic training
as it moves one into a level of awareness consistent
with that which brings about healing. Here are the
steps:

1. Relax the body, from the bottom to top or top
   to bottom.
2. Create a condition of mild warmth through
   the entire body.
3. Slow down the heart a bit. Bring about some
   cardiac regulation.
4. Slow down the breathing. This is a transition
   step, where one assumes the condition that
   "It breathes me." The awareness begins here
   to separate from the physical body. The consciousness and the physical body move away
   from each other.
5. Next, develop a state of abdominal warmth.
6. Create next a sensation of coolness in the
   forehead.

This, then, is the state of consciousness that has
been called the alpha state. Physical conditions can

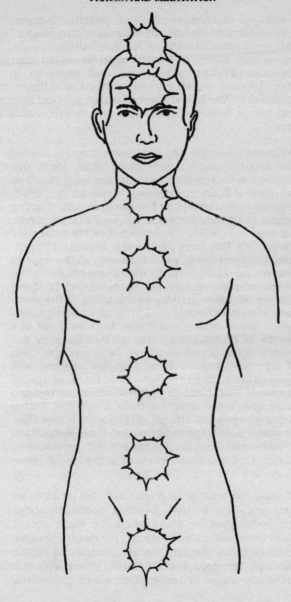

be repaired in this state—and psychic awareness can be enhanced by the utilization of this state. Dr. Jacob explored this idea in his workshop.

As various states of what might be called altered consciousness were discussed and explored to a degree, I found myself remembering the chapter on meditation in the Edgar Cayce *Search for God* books. There are a few excerpts that are worth quoting here:

> When we quiet the physical body through tuning the mind toward the highest ideal, there are aroused actual physical vibrations, as a result of spiritual influence becoming active on the sensitive vibratory centers in the body, stimulating the points of contact between the soul and its physical shell. . . . With the arousing of the image, or ideal, this life force (from the glands of reproduction) rises along what is known as the Appian Way or the silver cord, to the pineal center in the brain, whence it may be disseminated to those centers that give activity to the whole of the mental and physical being. . . . Thus on entering meditation there arises a definite impulse from the glands of reproduction that passes through the pineal to the pituitary gland. Whatever the ideal of an individual is, it is propelled upward and finds expression in the activity of the imaginative forces. If this ideal is material, there is builded more and more into the body a love for, and a tendency towards, things of the earth. If this ideal or image is of a spiritual nature, there is spiritual development. Psychic forces are only an awakening of soul faculties through activities in these centers.

> Cleanse the body with pure water. Sit or lie in an easy position, without binding garments about the body. Breathe in through the right nostril three times and exhale through the mouth. Breathe in three times through the left nostril and exhale through the right nostril. Then, either with the aid of low music or incantation which carries the

self deeper into a sense of oneness with the creative forces of love, enter into the Holy of Holies.
As self feels or experiences the rising of this, see it
disseminated through the inner eye (not carnal
eye) to that which will bring the greater understanding in meeting every condition in the experience of the body. Then, we may listen to the music
that is made as each center of the body responds
to the new creative force that is being disseminated, each through its own channel. We will find
that, little by little, meditation will enable us to
renew ourselves physically, mentally and spiritually.

Search for God Book II, pp. 129–30)

One does not usually think in terms of meditation
during the final stages of pregnancy, especially when
the onset of labor and leaking of amniotic fluid
occurs with still five weeks to go. But an A.R.E.
Clinic patient recently did in fact begin having labor
pains under such circumstances. She was seen in
the Clinic immediately, and Nitrazine paper tests
showed that nearly a pint of amniotic fluid had indeed escaped, and the patient was having regular
contractions of the uterus.

She was immediately admitted to Doctors Hospital
labor room, and a monitor was attached to record
uterine contractions and fetal heart rate. This is
where meditation came into the picture. The patient
and her husband had been meditating regularly for
more than a year, and her doctor suggested to her
that with meditation, she could possibly seal up
those membranes that were leaking and stop the
contractions. She went to work, along with her
husband, to quiet things down. When the Nitrazine
paper was used after the patient had been quiet for
nearly five fours, it was negative for amniotic fluid.

The importance of such an effect is obvious to the
obstetrician. Forty-eight hours of intramuscular medication at that point can mature the infant's lungs so
there would be little or no problem with hyaline
membrane disease if the child is then born prematurely. If delivery can be held off for that period of
time, there is the possibility that pregnancy can be

maintained for five weeks more. Then the baby has its greatest chance to be born fully normal. Many obstetricians try to hold off the contractions by giving the pregnant mother intravenous alcohol to relax the uterus. It does provide the necessary time to mature the infant's lungs, but it also intoxicates the mother and the child.

With meditation techniques applied successfully, alcohol can be avoided and the parents can grow spiritually by understanding in application that there are energies within the body that can be used constructively to bring about proper functions when they are desperately needed. In this instance, the mother meditated to bring about a quieting of the entire body. The uterine contractions stopped. Then she tried to visualize stopping the fluid from leaking through the membrances into the vagina. This was unsuccessful. Then she thought that perhaps the leaking membranes were higher in the uterus. So, in her mind, she began to spin a web around the inside of the uterus, from up near the top down to the area over the cervical opening. The leaking stopped.

Final result? One would hope for a continuation of pregnancy until the full nine months were accomplished. However, at least the forty-eight hours were fulfilled. Indeed, two days passed without labor, and a half-day beyond that. But the mother did deliver prematurely. The infant, however, with intramuscular medication, had time to mature its lungs, and there was no problem aside from the prematurity. The newborn prospered and was soon discharged to be home with its mother.

To sum up, both prayer and meditation should be part of each individual's daily activities. Through them, as Edgar Cayce pointed out in many readings, one can gain greater insights into oneself and therefore better balance and health—physically, mentally, and spiritually.

Chapter Thirteen
ATTITUDES AS AN
AID TO HEALING

Attitudes do not just happen! They are built by the mind, and they can be changed simply by recognizing that they are really under our direction and control—and by desiring deeply that they be changed. An attitude is like a direction. If one is headed toward New York from Kansas City but really wants to go to Los Angeles, he certainly must first recognize that he is headed east, and then he must turn around and take a new direction.

If a father constantly criticizes his teen-age daughter's schoolwork and her relationships with boyfriends, and at the same time he deeply desires the closeness of a loving father-daughter relationship, then he needs first to recognize that destructive criticism (and sometimes even constructive criticism) creates a distance in any relationship, not a deepening, closer walk together. Then, after recognizing that fact, he needs to do a turnaround and move off in a new direction, finding in her looks, her work, and her activities those wonderful talents that he tells her about. That creates the closeness. The recognition of the need and the subsequent action taken in a new direction are the two essential elements required for changing attitudes that may be causing stress and unhappiness.

When an individual takes even the most effective medication for a given illness, but his attitude is "that's not going to do me a bit of good!"—then he is not likely to get well. When one of my elderly patients lost his wife, I was concerned because he was so depressed and felt that life was useless for him. He developed a pneumonitis of the lungs, and although the bacteria were sensitive to a number of

antibiotics, no amount of the proper medication
stopped what became an overwhelming infection,
and the man died.

In the Cayce material, a variety of applications to
the physical body were recommended as being of
aid—including massage, diathermy, violet ray, the
ultraviolet lamp, and castor oil packs. But attitudes
that are constructive were always part of the whole
treatment and were never to be forgotten. In one
reading, Cayce said it like this:

> Let the attitude then be *constructive* ever! See in
> the applications taken not just rote, not just some-
> thing to be done, but—as the active force of every
> nature is God-influence work—creating in and
> through the individual—see with each applica-
> tion the creating of energies necessary for bring-
> ing cooperation with the service the Creator would
> have thee render in thine experience.
>
> For all become witnesses to His grace, His mercy,
> in the experiences of the activities in the material
> plane.
>
> 1424–1

Emotions and attitudes can hinder or enhance a
person's effectiveness in all sorts of situations. Thus,
the attitude that one chooses to wear affects not
only what sort of job he might hold and what sort of
life partner he might attract, but also determines to
some extent the physiological imbalances and thus
the disease syndromes present in his body. The
choices one makes, then, may indeed be important
relative to how one structures his personality.

Listen to what Benjamin Franklin, in his autobio-
graphy, had to say about pride. A friend pointed out
to him that at times he was overbearing and even
insolent. Franklin added humility to his list of virtues to be learned, and wrote:

> I cannot boast of much success in acquiring the
> *reality* of this virtue, but I had a good deal with
> regard to the *appearance* of it. I made it a rule to

forbear all direct contradiction to the sentiments of others, and all positive assertions of my own. I even forbade myself the use of every expression or word in the language that imported a fixed opinion, such as *certainly, undoubtedly,* etc., and I adopted instead of them: *I conceive; I apprehend;* or *I imagine a thing to be so and so,* or *it so appears to be at present.*

I soon found the advantage of this change in my manner; the conversations I engaged in went on more pleasantly. The modest way in which I proposed my opinions procured them a readier reception and less contradiction; I had less mortification when I was found to be in the wrong; and I more easily prevailed with others to give up their mistakes and join with me when I happened to be in the right.

Unfortunately, the attitude of humility is not much talked about today; and, with respect to the healing process, it is also unfortunate that the attitude of the patient is not generally considered of any importance and is rarely regarded as taking part in the healing itself.

Holistic patient care demands that the patient be considered, that he be looked at as aiding in the healing process, or as hindering it, depending on him and his attitudes as the focal point for the entire process. One of the Cayce readings points up this particular concept to a multiple sclerosis patient who apparently was "down in the mouth"—at least at the time the reading was given. Cayce described the problem as primarily glandular, but aggravated by subluxations in the lumbar area. But it was a very typical early case of multiple sclerosis in a twenty-eight-year-old male. Before any therapy was suggested, Cayce had this to say:

First in the mental attitude:

Do not allow hindrances—of not being as others— to cause too great a depressing effect upon the purposes, aims, hopes of the body. Know that the

author of life, the author of hope, even as in Him,
is able to bring that in thine own experience in
and through which ye may be the greater blessings to others, and contribute thus—daily—in thy
associations with others, a hope, and a glorifying
of his holy name.

                                                      2929—1

How does one inspire hope in the patient, if hope
is indeed a potent healing force? Can a physician
afford to be anything but warm, gentle, understanding, and helpful in his attitudes toward his patients,
if he expects to get consistent and healing results in
his therapy? It was the attitude of the Cayce material that always inspired people and continues to do
so—primarily, I think, because of the constructive
nature of the advice given, magnifying the virtues,
in a very real sense, and minimizing the faults. The
potential of the human being must always be stressed,
and the "patient" must always experience a real
change in consciousness if a healing is to come
about.

Attitudes, it seems to me, are the means by which
the creative mind trains the emotions, the glandular
centers of the body. Attitudes are consciously chosen,
despite the frequently held opinion—after an out-
burst of anger—that "that's just the way I am!" The
reason I am that way is because I created myself that
way. I chose an attitude of reacting, rejecting,
rebelling, of being angry when anyone disagreed with
me, and I practiced it. The activity became habitual,
like all human repetitive activities, and then, "that's
just the way I am."

The correction of attitudes can be found in the
Bible, but not under the title you'd expect. The correction factor is called "fruits of the Spirit," and it is
found in the book of Galatians in the New Testament.
The book was written by Paul, who urged the early
Christians to pay no attention to their lower nature,
but rather to practice these fruits of the Spirit.

Imagine what would happen in an angry man's
head if he chose to understand his opponent, to
forgive him, and to be patient with him instead of

killing him. Perhaps it is too much to ask people to
love one another, for that is what the fruits of the
Spirit are all about. But the point of it all is that
these attitudes that we carry around with us are
self-generated, self-perpetuated—but, as habitual,
emotional, glandular responses, they can still be re-
trained in the direction one wants to take them.
Again, if one finds himself heading for New York
when he wants to go to Los Angeles, he must turn
around and start moving in a new direction. It takes
thought, choice, and action.

The mind, however, seems to be building many
things for us all on its own, without being called
upon to do so. Perhaps we could call it the mind of
the emotions, for that is what appears to be in control most of the time. Sometimes, however, the imagination gets into the picture and someone creates an
attitude consistent with a happening that can only
be imagined. Some years ago I read an article in
Today's Health (August 1970) entitled "Stigmata: A
Matter of Mind or Miracle?" It centered in on the
phenomenon of bleeding that occurs in the same
locations of the body as those from which Jesus bled
while on the cross nearly two thousand years ago.
Stigmatics (350 of them by actual count), from the
time of St. Francis of Assisi in 1224 A.D. up to the
present-time story of Padre Pio, are discussed in an
interesting manner in this article. Padre Pio died
more than ten years ago, but in his lifetime he experienced stigmata. He is reported also to have levi-
tated frequently while he was saying Mass. Vatican
representatives were sent to investigate the reports.
Both the stigmata and the levitation were witnessed,
and there were no needles or strings attached.

The author of the article compared stigmatics to
autoerythrocyte sensitization cases, discussed the
similarities, and concluded that stigmatics are a
"combination of psychogenic bleeding and autoerythrocyte sensitization."* What bothers me is that

*In autoerythrocyte sensitization, the red blood cells
(erythrocytes) undergo a sensitization process automati-
cally and bleed spontaneously through the skin.

reporters of such events so often leave out important contributory data. For instance, if Padre Pio's bleeding was psychogenic in origin, for the most part, was this also the origin of his ability to levitate when he said Mass? Was St. Francis's communion with wild animals a product also of a psychogenic defect that brought about his stigmata? Are all visions the product of a disturbed mind? Are all the cures noted at Lourdes, all the healings at the Kuhlman services, psychologically induced changes? My question really is this: Why must we always look at the relationship between God and man as if only science can determine what has happened, and that in terms of a materialistic viewpoint that does not admit the existence of a Creator-God?

From the data that are available to us, even without the material in the Cayce readings, one does not need to be a genius to understand that the mind and the body are *one*, in all parts of this that we call a body, and that consciousness exists in all parts of our being. It seems much more reasonable to conclude that autoerythrocyte sensitization is the result of a state of consciousness in one type of person whose consciousness is centered upon his body to an undue degree; while the stigmatic has desired to share some of the pain that *another person* experienced, and, using his imagination, his consciousness is thus moved over toward the one who to him most symbolizes the reality of God in his life. Such phenomena are, I believe, caused by a difference in consciousness, different experiences in creative imagination, with the physical changes perhaps being the results of the consciousness present.

Attitudes of mind can create problems or can help in their solution—or both—in the opinion of the Edgar Cayce readings. One particular case history helps to elaborate on this idea. Case 3100 was a thirty-nine-year-old man who had Parkinson's disease. He had never married, he lived with his mother, and the two of them were inseparable. He asked for a reading, and the physical discourse turned out to be oriented toward the patient's mental and spiritual welfare. The man apparently drank a good deal and

talked a lot, perhaps not listening as often as he
should have. Cayce gave him suggestions about his
diet, including plain foods, raw vegetable salads,
fish, fowl, and lamb as the only meats, and no fried
foods. He suggested massage to the spine and electrotherapy through the use of a B battery and a
solution jar using gold chloride and silver nitrate
solutions alternately on the positive side of the circuit.

Cayce suggested that the cause of the disease was
"those elements of gold and silver . . . lacking in
those periods of gestation, which produced in the
first cycle of activity the inability of the glands to
create." He also suggested that these elements could
be introduced into the body in this manner so that
the physical well-being of the body might be improved and eventually brought to normal—although
such improvement "becomes questionable" in many
quarters.

However, Cayce devoted a major portion of this
reading to the spiritual welfare of this unfortunate
man, and his comments are interesting, especially
as they pertain to the ten-year period following the
reading.

For, while we find there are pathological disturbances, these in their very nature indicate a pre-
natal disposition. Thus, if there would be physical or material help, the body's first approach will
necessarily be study of self.

Not in that attitude, "I didn't cause it," and "I
wasn't the effect of being brought into the earth,"
neither in the commanding of someone else for
those attitudes or the lack of consideration before
the birth.

But rather consider that the self is being given an
opportunity, here and how,—if it will accept
same,—to interpret, to understand, and to be of
help not only to self but in contributing something to the welfare of others in all their stages of
development or seeking for physical, mental and
spiritual help.

. . . That there was the so-called *meriting* of this interpretation, this understanding for this soul-entity, is indicated by the soul's choice and use of this opportunity for entrance into material manifestation.

Then, as you chose it, as you needed it, DO interpret it properly.

. . . Use those abilities of the mind in such measures and manners as to be ever a contributing influence for the creating of peace, harmony, love, kindness, gentleness, hope, in the minds and in the hearts of all with whom you come in contact day by day.

These are the first prerequisites if you would find help.

If you cannot accept this, forget it all. Do not even begin.

3100—1

In the question period, the man asked why the right side of his jaw slipped out of place time after time. The answer was direct and strong: "Talking too much, and then this is a part of the advancement of this condition—when nothing has been done much about it!" In the second answer given, Cayce repeated his warning about the need for spiritual attitudes being changed and the usefulness being directed—and if this was not done, the material applications certainly should not be undertaken.

The man apparently did not change his direction or his attitudes. The various treatments he received were to no avail. The problem, apparently, was with his attitudes, and ten years after the reading, the man died of coronary thrombosis.

One of the most helpful attitudes is joyfulness. To laugh, to make someone else smile at least three times a day—this is one of the Cayce remedies I have always remembered. And the joyfulness at meals instead of arguments may mean a healthy stomach rather than ulcers and chronic bowel problems. Or high blood pressure. We try at home to keep all the

conversation happy and light at mealtimes, for when
people eat together, something special happens. I
remember the Bible story of Jesus, after the res-
urrection, walking with two disciples on the road to
Emmaus. They did not recognize him. But when
finally they sat down and broke bread together, they
knew then that it was the Master.

We don't have that kind of experience today, but
we never know when we will be entertaining angels
unaware—so we keep our dinner-table conversation
creative, happy, and joyful.

Sickness often arises, however, out of the contro-
versies, the arguments, the sometimes ravishing
disharmonies that occur in the home. Karmic influences seem to draw together those who have problems within themselves to solve, and frequently this
is true between father and son. One father who had
such an opportunity to face was my patient many
years ago. He was in constant conflict with his son
who did not want to follow the profession his dad had
been in for years. The sickness here ended up as an
apparent complete shutdown of the adrenal glands,
and the father died as a result. However, it is interesting to reflect on the fact that, prior to his death—
a matter of less than two months—the father and son
had buried the hatchet, had come to a peaceful conclusion in their arguments, and had become good
friends. Perhaps this solution was the father's
primary goal this lifetime. It is difficult to say.

The home, however, was seen in the Cayce readings not as a place in which conflict should be the
manner of solving difficulties. Rather, Cayce said:

> The home is the nearest pattern in earth (where
> there is unity of purpose in the companionship)
> to man's relationship to his Maker.
>
> 3577-1

> And if each entity would so live in this material
> sojourn as if it were for an eternal home, much
> more beauty, much more joy, much more peace
> would be attained.
>
> 1872-1

Another father, who wishes to remain anonymous, found this kind of information in the readings to be a real factor in his life, and composed a letter to his eldest son that not only reflected how he felt his relationship to his son should be, but formed a pattern that created between the two a bond that he feels will last as long as these creative, constructive bonds should last—and I'm sure that involves many incarnations. He gave me permission to share this letter so that it might be helpful in counseling with those fathers and sons who are having difficulties that eventually will result in illness of the physical body, if not set at rest.

My Son:
There are but three gifts I would offer you, for the treasures of this world that you might want, most often must be gained only through long and sometimes bitter struggle. My gifts are free.

This first gift is only a concept, but I give it freely and ask only that you remember it and keep it deep within your heart: You are part God, for God is within you. Therefore, think in a Godly manner and act as God would have you act.

This also I would offer as a gift: Nothing is truth for you until you have proved it. Thus it is good that you think on all good things, and, when you have proved a truth by living it, add it unto yourself. In this way you will grow in stature.

The third gift, which, like the others, is only yours if you enter it into the ledger of your mind: Think! Remove all barriers from about the mind which would restrict the workings of that most wonderful ability each of us has received from God. Unless you do this, how then can you become more God-like?

Remember these things, my son, and my gifts to you will live forever within your own being, and with your growth I will grow likewise.

This father recognized that his growth really comes about when he is helpful in the growth process of another—in this instance, his son. The attitude of helpfulness, of hopefulness, the attitude of keeping an open mind and knowing that all things are possible—all these contribute toward one's health and aid in overcoming illness.

Illness, it seems to me, often is like a pitfall into which one stumbles in the darkness of night. For the illness actually does come from our lack of awareness of where our activities or emotions and attitudes are taking us—or else sometimes we simply don't care.

So it is important to assess our own attitudes. See if they are contributory to our illnesses. Better yet, appraise within our own selves what attitudes we want to develop that are constructive and that build health and a vigorous body balance. Then we need to act, for action makes it real, and in this way our healing progresses.

Chapter Fourteen
DREAMS IN HEALTH AND HEALING

Over the centuries of man's existence on Earth, dreams have been a constant companion to him in his hours of sleep, bringing information, guidance, self-knowledge, and communication from other dimensions of life. In the Old Testament, dreams saved Joseph's life in Egypt, led him into leadership, and through him provided a destiny for God's Chosen People. Similarly, in the New Testament, it was through a dream that Mary was told to give her unborn child the name of Jesus; and it was through a dream that Joseph and Mary were directed to flee to Egypt.

Early in the twentieth century, the studies of the great psychiatrists, Freud and Jung, brought more understanding than ever before to the nature of dreams. More recently, dreams have been studied in

the laboratory, and much has been learned about
their frequency—probably seven or more each night—
and the levels of sleep during which they occur.
Many books have been written about dreams, and
many observers of the dream state have recognized
that dreams give a wealth of information and in-
sight about the body itself, its state of health, and
what may need to be done to improve the body's
health. Notice of impending death is a common dream
subject; while, on the other hand, actual healings
can come spontaneously during a dream.

Dreams that are significant of the body's state of
health, of what the future holds in store for us, or of
what we should be doing are common events in
everyone's experience. Sometimes the story is simple and clear and needs no interpretation. At other
times, the symbology of the dream must be studied
and interpreted before its meaning becomes clear.
And still other dreams seem to be simply the result
of an unwise choice of dinner or a disturbed frame
of mind before retiring.

In my own experience, I have had all kinds of
dreams and have recorded them so that they will be
available for me to study. As a physician, I have
worked with my patients in unraveling the threads
of some of their difficult but important dreams, and
it has always been helpful. We frequently challenge
our patients to dream about the physician within
their own beings and to get his suggestions. For
within each person's body is the knowledge of what
is wrong when one is ill, and what most likely needs
to be done in order to get well.

One patient, who told me about his experiences,
had been plagued for months with a severely dis-
abling bursitis and had gained no relief from the
various treatments of a series of physicians. Then
he started reading about karma and how it shows
up in various physical problems. He went to sleep
one night and in a dream—or a vision—he asked:
"Is this condition karmic in origin?" There came a
voice in answer: "No—lift up your arms!" At that
point he woke and found both his arms lifted high
over his head, a position he had been unable to

assume consciously for months. He has had no problem with the bursitis since.

Dreams of this kind, while not commonplace, are not rare. All kinds of dreams take place every night in each person's experience, and—if they are heeded—they will give the dreamer help in times of trouble and inspiration when he is trying to be of service.

The Edgar Cayce material is a rich source for the understanding and utilization of dreams. During the course of Edgar Cayce's lifetime, there were more than nine hundred dream readings given. On several occasions, Cayce even recalled to the dreamer's mind the details of the dream that, in his conscious state, the dreamer had forgotten.

To one individual, on three different occasions, were given suggestions as to the meaning and use of dreams:

> . . . The dreams as we see come to the entity in those forms of the physical, of the spiritual, of the subconscious, and when studied aright may gain the more perfect knowledge concerning manifested forces of that creative force in a physical world.
>
> 136—16

> . . . The dreams as come to the body are those correlations of physical conditions through the body-mind, with the subconscious forces of the entity, and these may be developed to that point where the subconscious will give the directing way, through suggestions to same in the subjugated state of consciousness, see?
>
> 136—18

> . . . These [dreams], as we see, are those conditions which have come to the mental development of the entity from time to time. They may be applied, may be made applicable in the daily life of the entity.
>
> 136—21

In his readings, Cayce also stated that sometimes it is difficult for us to differentiate between dreams and visions, for we probably have both coming to us for our enlightenment—if we will but accept it. He also spoke of the dream sense as a sixth sense—a greater ability within us for our adventure here in this plane of consciousness that we call Earth.

In working with dreams, it is helpful to work with a group. Finding meaning to one's dreams is hard work. It takes time; it takes discipline in recording them; and it takes practice to analyze them.

Some Dreams

"Big old house" dreams came to be the title of a series of emblematic material presented to the sleeping-waking consciousness of one of my patients some fifteen to twenty years ago. She tells part of the story herself:

> In the last twenty years or more I have been dreaming of big old houses with large rooms, all of these in an extreme disorder and messed up. Each house had a number of oversized rooms— many, many rooms. And no matter what the type of house it was in the dream, the house seemed to be familiar to me and was my house.
>
> The rooms sometimes had knocked-out walls, or very dirty walls. The rugs had holes in them and the furniture was out of place. The floor had holes in it, and in general the house was always in a mess.
>
> I was willing to clean up my house in every dream, but it all looked so difficult and hopeless and impossible that I just stood in the middle of the room with an extremely depressed feeling, not knowing how to straighten up my house and feeling very helpless.
>
> When I awoke from these dreams, it sometimes took me ten minutes to realize that it was only a dream, but the depressed feeling still persisted for at least two hours after the dream was ended and I awoke. It seemed to me, every time I had one of these "messed up house" dreams that I was in a very deep sleep.
>
> Since I joined the A.R.E. in the fall of 1963, I

stopped having dreams of these old houses. This
was in October 1963, when I became a study-
group member.

Instead, in January 1964, I had a dream of a
house not quite as large as the ones I always
dreamed of before, but it seemed to be a normally
sized house. I just finished, in the dream, with
papering one room with a wallpaper that was beige
in color and had a green border. I also had purchased two large cans of paint for another room.

Obviously, these cans of paint signified a new beginning for the dreamer, for she continued painting
her house in subsequent dreams, and the house
became larger and more beautiful, until several years
later she drove up to her house and found it was a
mansion, worth millions of dollars. She had other
dreams, of course, dealing with troubles in the
fireplace, occasional smoke in the house, etc., but
the direction of the dreaming was constructive, joyful,
and hopeful. One doesn't need much dream-inter-
pretation ability to recognize the dramatic change
that took place in the awareness, the consciousness,
and the lifestyle of the dreamer during the course of
that simple series of dreams.

Doctors' appointments in the New Age sometimes
come about in the most unusual manner. We have a
friend who wanted to see a dentist in the Scottsdale
area here in Arizona. In a dream she saw the dentist's
name on the door of his office. She woke up and
looked up the name in the phone book—and sure
enough, there it was, right in Scottsdale. She made
an appointment, and on her information sheet she
put down that she had been referred by a dream.

One story like that is not enough. Some time ago
Dr. Gladys McGarey saw a woman in her office and
happened to ask her how she had come to the Clinic.
The story emerged: She had a dream that awakened
her in the middle of the night. She heard the name
McGarey. Before she had gone to sleep she had been
wondering what she could do about getting guidance for her health. She went back to sleep and
twice more was awakened by a dream. Each time

the words came, "McGarey can help—McGarey can
help."

In the morning, she asked her husband if he knew
anyone by that name. He did not. That night, she
went to a movie with a friend, and during the course
of the evening she asked her if she knew anyone by
the name of McGarey. Her friend responded: "Sure.
They're doctors at the A.R.E. Clinic." A phone call
was made, the appointment was secured, and on
the information sheet she wrote (because she was a
bit hesitant) not that a dream had referred her but
rather "a friend." Dreams can be friendly, too!

In teaching others to care for themselves in a holistic manner, the dream state cannot be ignored.
Through dreams come advice, assistance, and guidance for the physical body as well as for the individual as a whole. One of my patients recently brought
me an interesting dream. She is being treated for
arthritis along the lines suggested in the Cayce
readings, and she also has had consistent problems
with eliminations. I saw her and discussed the dream
with her some ten days after she had recorded it.
Here is her dream:

> I dreamt I was cleaning house, when I picked up
> the toilet-brush holder and removed the brush,
> and noticed that one of the brushes was broken.
> It was still usable and I considered keeping it
> until I could replace it, but then decided it could
> not do a thorough job, so threw it away.

On awakening from the dream, the woman knew
that the dream referred to her body and also that
she had a rash on her back. Nothing in the dream
had said that, but she *knew* a rash was there. So
she looked in the mirror—but there was no rash.
She couldn't dispel the idea, and the next day when
she went back for a therapy treatment, she asked
the therapist to check her back for a rash. There
was no trace of a rash. When the therapist asked
what kind of rash she was expecting, she said, "Like
the spot on my leg." That particular spot had been
there for several days. Then, over the course of the

next three days, a rash did in fact develop over her back, which brought her to the Clinic a week after the dream. I made the diagnosis of pityriasis rosea. Interesting dream contact, isn't it, drawing precognitive physical information from the unconscious mind, which obviously must have had it. And the dream itself spoke of problems with eliminations and the cleansing of the body.

One night, another of my patients had a craving for fruit, and he ate a whole quart of canned pears just before going to bed. The following dream came to him that night: "I was on a fishing boat that was hindered in its progress because the pilot had carelessly atttempted to go right through a thick bed of kelp." He woke up, needing bathroom privileges quite badly. When he started recording the dream, it occurred to him that the botanical name of kelp is *macrocystis pyrifera*—which means "pear-bearing large bladder."

Apparently, his dream was telling him what he already knew—that he had overeaten a single food item before retiring. But it also told him that his "fishing trip"—what might be called his spiritual quest in the dream state—was rather foolishly held up through his eating habits. Also, he learned that pears, for him certainly, at least in the canned form, would have an active influence on his bladder, so beware.

Other Dimensions

Edgar Cayce implied that in one sense we are more alive in the dream state than while walking around in the physical dimension that some have called the world of duality. This fits in with the religious belief that we are basically spiritual creatures and that our normal habitat is a spiritual one, not material. Sometimes, individuals will move in a state of extended consciousness to touch what has been called the Akashic records. Some see it as a tapestry that each individual weaves with every thought and feeling and action in this world of experience. Some see it as a book for each person in

a large, large library, of sorts. It appears that the
Akasha can be understood in any way that makes
three-dimensional sense to the person who locates
it. It is important to tell what has been discovered to
others who may understand it only in terms of this
world. Even Cayce saw the Akasha in different ways
during his lifetime.

Such a concept reminds me of a dream given to
me some time ago that was related by a ten-year-old
girl to her mother, but which was so impressive to
the girl that it persisted in her memory vividly from
that point onward. But it tells how this young girl
perceived something that obviously was other-dimen-
sional, while at the same time it had to be understandable to a ten-year-old mind:

> When I was nine or ten years old, I had my tonsils
> and adenoids removed. While under the anesthe-
> sia I could hear the cells in my body talking to one
> another. They were all very busy doing their ap-
> pointed duties. One group would say to another,
> "This is as far as we go, now you take over, etc."
> This was going on all over my body and I seemed
> to be listening to it. So much activity, each doing
> their appointed work and content in it. As I lis-
> tened to all this I thought, "This must be how life
> begins and a body is formed and that each cell
> has intelligence and an appointed task to perform."
> I've thought of this dream often through life.

When one considers that cells have been grown in
cultures to create miniature functioning cell systems of the brain, the heart, and other organs, and
when one realizes that the Peyer's patches produce
cells with a fantastic memory, one begins to compre-
hend that cells have consciousness of a sort, being
able to develop toward a goal and to have the power
of memory. Cayce apparently communicated with
the body, or the consciousness of the body, when he
gave a reading, so it might be understandable that
the cells might have a language that can be interpreted
by the dream faculty as speech. We are indeed more
wonderful than we are wont to believe!

The passing over of a loved one is often perceived in a dream, even long before it happens. It seems never to be death itself that is seen in the dream. When one dies in a dream, it is usually symbolic of new awareness coming into being; for it really is dying to one reality of consciousness and being born into another. So, death in a dream understandably means new life.

A good friend of mine recently described his dreams about his mother. They were walking up a shaded path that was beautiful with flowers and trees lining the pathway. They came to a place where the path divided into two. His mother wanted to go to the right with her son, but she told him she had to take the path to the left. This was one of a series of similar dreams that preceded her death by several months.

Death of the physical body is also predicted when it seems hardly reasonable to the conscious waking mind. This happened to a family who are both friends and patients. The husband, who has a long history of heart disease, had refused to come in for evaluation of his heart condition, insisting to his wife, just the night of his demise, that "this is my heart." Just a week prior to the heart attack that brought about his death, his wife had a dream. The two of them were walking down a road that stretched out a long way. There was another road that branched off to the left a little way ahead, and before they would come to the branching of the road there was a bridge that crossed over a stream, also to the left.

A little building stood beside the bridge. The two were arguing. He wanted to cross over the bridge, and she wanted to take the road that branched off to the left. It was straight, also, well paved, and she was sure it was right. She went into the little building and found a jolly, heavyset woman there who volunteered the information that the road chosen by the dreamer was correct. Then she looked at the bridge and saw wispy, wavy figures, ill defined, weaving and moving in the middle of the bridge. Very difficult to define. She felt apprehensive about her husband, and went to look for him, but couldn't find him. The dream ended there.

It was less than a week after the dream that the heart attack came. I'm sure the unconscious mind of the wife got the message, but consciously she wasn't sure about the meaning of the dream until I discussed it with her several weeks later. She understood the spiritual implications of life and the importance of dreams, so it was a helpful event in her life to know that it was by choice that her husband had left.

Dreams will always remain a source of information, guidance, and aid, not only to the interested observer but to the one who seeks help in his physical condition. For the physical, the mental, and the spiritual are really one, and we need all the help we can get to keep the part of us well that we can see and feel—although we still cannot really understand its total working.

Chapter Fifteen
PUTTING IT ALL TOGETHER

When we start to put things together—the concepts, the nature of man, what healing really is, the tools, the methods—we should begin to look at our goal as a process. Healing is never really an instantaneous thing. There are cells in our body dying every moment, and new cells being born. We are constantly in a state of change, and we should understand that it may take seven years for all the atoms to be changed in our bodies. If atoms have consciousness, as Edgar Cayce suggested, then our consciousness can undergo a total change in those seven years. Healing, then, becomes a change in our physical, our mental, and our spiritual beings, and that change is a process that happens over a span of time.

Most of us don't want to wait to have something corrected. We want the surgeon to remove it or the plastic surgeon to correct it. Or we want the antibiotic to destroy the bacteria. If we are successful, we may have gained much. On the other hand, we may not have learned what patience is, and we may not have understood that we need to learn patience. For, as the readings so frequently indicate, our souls demand patience. It is the third dimension of space and time in which we do our work.

We also have difficulty in seeing changes occur when we are doing the monitoring ourselves. We become anxious when it appears that a condition is worsening, and these anxieties are, in themselves, a barrier to the healing process. And then we also confront the question of karma and its apparently unbeatable formula: as you sow, so shall you reap. We find ourselves asking which conditions are karmic, and if they can indeed by overcome.

To be successful in working with this wonderful organism that we call the human body, however, we need to keep a perspective of patient observation of what is happening, remembering that the body is capable of regeneration, that hope and prayers, meditation, good nutrition, exercise, massage, dreams, and simple therapies all lend their impact on the body and lead toward a state of health. Directions need to be remembered.

In the process of caring for ourselves, in putting it all together, we will be unsuccessful from time to time and have to make a trip to our doctor's office. Nevertheless, it would be well to remember that we have a right to be heard with regard to our own health.* We have something significant to say about our own health and welfare, and we should say it.

Working with the maintenance of life and the creation of health where disease once existed is the central focus of this book. Preventive care—the things one should do to keep illness away—is the key. Of interest to those concerned with prevention is the manner in which the information from the Edgar

*This right is pointed up dramatically in the book *Between Doctor and Patient*, by Donald M. Hayes, M.D. (Valley Forge, PA: Judson Press, 1977).

Cayce readings is used by members of the A.R.E. and by patients of the numerous doctors who follow the concepts in the readings. We have received literally thousands of letters from individuals who have used the ideas in the readings for care of illness and, more especially, for prevention of illness. For the thrust of the readings leads one to a lifestyle that is preventive of illness by its very nature:

> For, all healing comes from the One Source. And, whether there is the application of foods, exercise, medicine or even the knife—it is to bring [to] the consciousness of the forces within the body, that aid in reproducing themselves [which is] the awareness of Creative or God Forces.

> 2696-1

Certainly, if the awareness of Creative Forces is the healing element in exercise or foods or medicine or surgery, then certainly anything that will bring that awareness to the body *prior* to the onset of any disease process will prevent it. And, indeed, it is the unawareness, the lack of consciousness of the Divine, that in the final analysis is the cause of disease, as the essential story unfolds in the Cayce readings.

New Age Medicine

Physicians who find themselves in the midst of New Age medicine are having a hard time of it, for they find their patients starting to care for themselves in a creative manner. But also they find practical issues revolving around the *right* of those same people to choose the kind of treatment they want or think they should have. The right to choose is a political "hot potato." To what extent should the medical professional intrude upon people to protect them? Deeply involved in such a question is what should be done about practitioners who use some of the most controversial treatments in health care: laetrile for cancer, chelation therapy for hardening of the arteries, and bee stings for arthritis.

The question of right or wrong cannot be judged

simply on the scientific merits of the treatments under consideration. Factors other than scientific validity also need to be considered. Dr. John Bunker, a physician and Standford University Medical School faculty member, has pointed out that even scientific questions are not easily resolved. "One-third to one-half of what physicians do is based on poor evidence or no evidence," he said, "and the data is often imperfect or contradictory." He added that researchers "often fit the data to fit their own conceptions. . . . We are all biased." Dr. Bunker himself felt that, when experts disagree on a subject, "it seems appropriate to let the public make up its own mind." Yet, at the same time, he felt that there is an obligation to protect the public from the greatest abuses, since the sea of uncertainty is an invitation to quackery, and it is too much to expect the public to make the "horrendous" decisions by themselves.

There will be trouble in dealing with these issues until spiritually based concepts get infused into the decision-making to the degree that individuals are recognized for what they really are—spiritual beings created in the image of the Creator, with an unlimited capacity to understand, to choose, and to become more and more in the image of that which brought them into being.

The methods suggested in the Cayce readings for the prevention and correction of illnesses are aimed at improving function of the body and the mind, while most therapies are really aimed at diseases, not recognizing that the diseases are really products of improper, confused physiological functions. And the physical body certainly has the ability to regenerate. This has been dealt with earlier, but it should be brought to mind again. Cayce said it like this:

One should consider, as in this body, that the physical body in its creation was and is given the ability to reproduce itself. Thus each organ, each portion of the body secretes, from the physical, the mental and the spiritual life, that needed to reproduce itself for a growth to better conditions— or the realm for which it prepares itself. When

these activities break down, these have to be supplied or they call on other portions of the organism—and thus they become overcharged or
under-nourished. Then disintegration begins in
one form or another.

3337–1

When that disintegration has become a fact, and
the body is given influences to bring it back to
normal, there is often a feeling of discouragement
and frustration, because healing is not coming about
as quickly as has been desired. One wonders if in
fact there is really anything going on that is helpful
or creative. The message, for those of us who are
putting it all together, is simply: "Don't get discour-
aged or overanxious." Much harm can come to the
healing process if this comes about, for those emotions can create havoc within the body.

Do not become overanxious—for, to be sure, the
Mental is the Builder; and overanxiousness may
bring about barriers to proper reactions throughout the system; whether as related to the circulatory forces or the assimilations or eliminations of
the body.

But these influences kept in a body—normal
eliminations, near to normal assimilations—without accident—it, the body, reproduces itself in
every phase of its experience. . . .Keep these physically, mentally, with a spiritual basis of construc-
tiveness for the mental attitudes. For grudges,
animosities, hates, overanxieties are a part of the
mental and become conditions reactory in the
physical forces.

818–9

When one is faced with a serious illness, a chronic
illness, and is given a course of therapy to follow—
therapy designed to alter and upgrade the functions
of the body—he may suspect that the condition,
responding so slowly if at all, is a karmic one. Knowing about karma helps, because it gives one the

perspective of reincarnation and the possibility of another lifetime where his problems will have been set at rest. But the question always persists: "Can I get over it?" I learned a long time ago that almost any condition can be corrected; and that the law of karma is reversible through the law of grace, or forgiveness. Cayce once said that "the law of cause and effect is immutable *by choice.*" This means, of course, that deep within ourselves we can choose either to be healed or to live through this thing, because it may be the only way that we, with our obstinacy and our hard heads, can learn the lesson that the schoolteacher is giving us.

Putting it all together certainly means several things. I don't think we will ever be without the need for doctors and their expertise learned through many years of intensive study. But we all are creative, and we all have all knowledge locked deep within our own beings. So we should not shortchange ourselves. We should be able to give ourselves sufficient credence that we can approach the upgrading of our bodies with a degree of assurance and great expectations.

We might keep these two extracts from the Cayce readings in mind as we work with our bodies and our minds:

Find thy ideals in spiritual things—then those in the mental and material will be the result.

Build . . . rather upon those things that are as eternal influences in the experience; and these will bring harmony where there have been turmoils heretofore.

2284—1

For, to heal a body-physical and not give it hope in the spiritual is to save a body for destruction in materiality.

518—1

Let's keep that hope alive in our spiritual nature, as we seek to upgrade the health of our country by bringing healing to ourselves in body, mind, and spirit. Let's go through the process of realizing what healing is all about—what health really is; let's remember that regeneration is always a possibility; let's maintain a constructive diet and a good exercise program; let's be creative about establishing helpful attitudes. Let's look into the inner side of our beings through our dreams, and let's continue a strong pattern of prayer and meditation. Then, let's add the other aids that may be needed for our present state of being.

Part Three
A FUNCTIONAL APPROACH TO THE BODY

Chapter Sixteen

AN INTRODUCTION TO FUNCTIONS AND SYSTEMS

Part 3 will be arranged according to functions and systems of the body that have begun to act improperly. The therapy indicated will be directed toward restoration of normal function to the affected area. Sometimes, such as in the problems of assimilation and elimination, organs or systems of the body will be identified as chapter titles. There are two organs of assimilation working in our bodies—the lungs and the upper intestinal tract; and four channels of elimination—the skin, the lungs, the kidneys, and the liver-intestinal tract. In these chapters there will inevitably be overlapping to some extent; however, it will be the *function* rather than the organ itself that will be stressed.

It is up to the reader to identify where his or her troubles may lie, for whatever help that may come from this book will only come in *application* as the body is brought to a better balance, as more coordination is achieved in the functioning of one's organism as a whole, and as awareness of the Divine within grows, for that spells health as well as alleviation of disease and healing. Remember, the body *is* the temple of the Living God.

As an aid, here is a checklist to use to begin any health-building program for yourself or a loved one. It should be a basic part of every therapy program in order to get the most out of your efforts.

1. Have you identified yourself as a spiritual being?
2. Have you recognized that regeneration is possible?
3. Have you started a diet that is helpful to you?

4. Have you begun a regular exercise program?
5. Have you established a regular period for prayer and meditation? And asked others to pray for you?
6. Have you started developing creative and positive attitudes and emotions?
7. Have you sought guidance through dreams?
8. Have you used any creative visualization techniques?

Adding to this the specifics from the following chapters and your own individual nature, let us then begin to put it all together!

Chapter Seventeen
THE LUNGS AND RESPIRATION

Each breath taken into the human body changes that body in a way that we do not fully understand. Oxygen is taken into the alveoli or small air sacs of the lungs, where it comes in close contact with minute blood cells or pulmonary capillaries; it is then picked up by the bloodstream in a chemical combination called oxyhemoglobin, and carried to all parts of the body, thereby keeping all our cells alive. We cannot live more than a few minutes without breathing air and its most important constituent, oxygen. Other, more subtle substances also come into the body through the air we breathe, aiding the body in less remarkable, yet important, ways.

The lungs and the respiratory tract must be classified, then, as part of those organs of the body that contribute to the life-giving function that we call assimilation—the ingesting, transforming, and utilizing of substances that are important for cellular function and reproduction.

In exchange for oxygen, the lungs provide the mechanism for removing from the bloodstream substances that are called metabolites—Edgar Cayce calls them "used and refused forces." These metabolites are the end products, principally carbon dioxide, excreted by the lung, which are breathed out when oxygen is breathed in. Other, less defined substances are also removed from the blood.

Thus, in further clarifying the function of the respiratory tract taken as a whole, we must grant it status also as an eliminatory organ. It helps remove from the body substances that, if left there, would act as toxins to all the tissues. The lungs, then, are one part of what we call the eliminatory system of the body—the others being the skin, the kidneys, and the combined liver-intestinal tract.

As part of the respiratory function, in addition to the lungs themselves, we have: the bronchi, the trachea, the larynx, the pharynx, the mouth, the nose, and the sinuses. All these structures reflect the body's wisdom to define structure according to required function. The microscopic, hairlike cilia that line the walls of the trachea or "windpipe" and its two branches (bronchi) move foreign substances upward so that they might be discharged through the mouth, thus aiding in the general housecleaning of this area of the body.

Any part of the respiratory tract can be affected by its environment, thereby improving or injuring its function. The nervous system, through spontaneous incoordination, may create confusion throughout the muscles and active parts of the system. Or the nerves may work in harmony with one another. Again, the bloodstream may be hampered in its flow or contain injurious substances; or the white blood cells, which are part of the normal constituency of the blood, may not function up to par for any number of reasons, allowing the onset of difficulties that are then called diseases. Still again, the air we breathe may be loaded with noxious substances that further disturb cellular function or cause actual pathological damage.

The cellular components of respiration respond as best they can under all circumstances; but if there are too many disturbing and destructive influences, illness results, and literally hundreds of diseases are associated with the structures that support the function of breathing.

From the standpoint of viewing function as the most important consideration, rather than the name of a disease, one must carry out certain therapeutic measures to enhance functions that may be performing inadequately. As these measures are applied in a balanced effort, a general response is elicited, and frequently that is all that is needed to restore normal function. My secretary, for instance, finds that by following a diet that excludes most sweets and starches during a time of high allergens in the air, her allergies improve. While it will take more than a diet to correct the allergic condition permanently, a start has been made.

Therapy for respiratory problems can be aimed initially at restoring general functions, and then specifics can be added as seems appropriate. A basic diet probably establishes the foundation of sound therapy for any part of this system. Diet in most cases would aim to eliminate sweets, white sugar or white flour, and all fried foods, be low on starches, and be high in fruits and vegetables (fresh and cooked). Fish, fowl, and lamb would be best in providing proteins. Rest is an important component of therapy, as well as the avoidance of excess emotional stress. Manipulative treatments or massages, especially to the upper part of the back, would generally be helpful, as would the use of an inhalant. Body eliminations should be encouraged.

Thus, the five basics in a therapy program are: (1) diet; (2) rest; (3) manipulative treatments; (4) inhalants; and (5) enhanced eliminations.

Elimination is closely related to diet. In the Cayce readings there is a vital concept of physiology not discussed to any extent in the textbooks—namely, that assimilation and elimination need to be balanced for health to occur. This means that all the activities involved in taking food into the body and utilizing it in body-building metabolic processes need to be looked at in relationship to how the body rids itself of wastes. As was indicated previously, elimination is accomplished by the lungs, the skin, the liver and intestinal tract, and the kidneys. According to Cayce, each of these four channels of elimination must be balanced in their individual activity as well as properly balanced as a unit when compared with assimilations.

In my own experience with the Cayce readings as they apply to common respiratory ailments, I have found that there are a multitude of ways to help clear up such problems, all apparently relating to the idea of establishing balance within the system. Most infections of this part of the body are associated with overacidity of the tissues; and frequently simply restoring a normal alkaline balance will allow the cells of the body to conquer the infectious organisms.

Jim, one of my foreign correspondents, found reality in this concept. Coming home from a four-day business trip with a full-blown cold and also what he called the flu, he had three things happen almost simultaneously: he remembered an article in the *A.R.E. News*, "Balance—The End to the Common Cold"; a member of his study group told him about using baking soda in hot water to help him out of the cold; and then a long-distance phone call from his mother reminded him that she, too, had always recommended baking soda in hot water for the common cold.

Jim took ½ teaspoon of baking soda in a large mug of hot water and sipped it slowly until gone. He did this once every hour until he went to bed, consuming by that time five mugs of water and 2½ teaspoons of baking soda. The next day, upon awakening, he started again with a mugful of soda water every two hours. He had lots of fluids and orange juice that day. That evening he went to a meeting. He had no more cold, no more flu, but he was still weak. The third day, he worked half a day, taking soda water in the morning and evening. Finally, on the fourth day, Jim felt great and was fully up to par.

But the strangest thing that happened to Jim was the least expected. For four months he had been sorely distressed by excessive sweating throughout the area of the groin, improper urination, incomplete emptying of the bladder, and "spasmodic" urination. And sometimes his need to urinate was so urgent that he would wet his pants before he could get to the bathroom. In fact, he would always carry a change of underwear and another pair of pants with him for such emergency.

Now, four months later, while experiencing the exhilaration of recovery from a severe cold, he realized that all these urinary troubles had completely disappeared. In the six months that followed, there was no recurrence. Balance! Cayce said in his readings that with proper alkaline balance, one could not get a cold. But Jim discovered that there are other advantages to be derived from a balanced body.

In one of his readings (8–2), Cayce suggested to a woman subject to colds that she alternate using Glycothymoline and Listerine mouthwash, swallowing the bit that was left after expelling the major portion. She was then to take Alophen 1/80 grain each week, while also getting osteopathic manipulations. All of this was aimed at helping her to obtain balance.

Most of the people I see are beyond the limits of just the cold itself. They usually have a degree of secondary infection, feel more than just a little bit miserable, and are at the point of having to miss work. So I suggest that they cleanse their bodies, increase the circulation, achieve a more normal acid-base balance, and gently stimulate the involved cells toward a higher function while letting the body rest more. Now, these varying degrees of physiological assistance *might* be instigated through the medium of self-suggestion—no question about this. However, I find this a difficult medium to work with and rely on the more physical means that the general practitioner finds readily available. So, I give them the following routine:

(1) One teaspoon each of *salt and soda* enema to warm water.

(2) A *hot bath* until perspiring, followed by a brisk rubdown in the bathroom to avoid getting chilled. Then *massage* into the chest, neck, and feet a solu-

tion made of equal parts of mutton tallow, spirits of turpentine, and spirits of camphor, mixing the materials in the order named. Then go to bed bundled up well for two hours, and in the next few days get lots of rest.

(3) A *diet* of fruit and fruit juices for the first twenty-four hours, with lots of water, then gradually add vegetables, light foods, meat, and then starches, but slowly, over the next few days. A light diet is essential, and the fruits and vegetables will act as one would suspect of alkaline-reacting foods. A general vitamin tablet with each meal for a few days supports the body during this time of stress.

(4) One teaspoon of an *inhalant* placed in an old two-pound coffee can, filled to about one-third full with boiling water. The fumes from this are inhaled through an inverted paper funnel placed over the can until all the fumes are exhausted. The inhalant is made up as follows:

Oil of eucalyptus	90 minims/drops
Rectified oil of turpentine	30 minims/drops
Oil of pine needles	5 minims/drops
Tolu in solution	5 minims/drops
Compound tincture of benzoin	110 minims/drops

As Edgar Cayce indicated, the inhalant acts as a cleanser for the cells lining the respiratory tract, so that they might act more normally. Not only does it clear up the cough almost always, it frequently aids the resolution of the infection. Beyond this, however, it gives the patient something to do that is creative for him as an individual, knowing that he is contributing to his own healing process—far better than just taking a pill.

While this procedure undoubtedly will not cure one hundred percent of all colds, it will make believers out of the great majority. One might think: How in the world can such a simple group of things do *anything* for a cold? By giving the body sufficient assistance, you regain health, and in a healthy body a cold just cannot exist. It is just about that simple.

Cayce's suggestions and therapies for alleviation of the common cold and accompanying cough are many. For case 585, Cayce suggested Sal Hepatica, three doses, two hours apart; to be followed by one-half teaspoon of Castoria every hour until the digestive tract was cleared. This same individual was told to treat his fever by bathing his feet in hot water every four hours, and, following this, to take a rub-down from the hips to the feet and including the feet with the combination already mentioned of equal parts of mutton tallow, spirits of turpentine, and spirits of camphor, put together in that order.

Such a combination was also suggested at times to be used on the throat and chest and over the sinuses—but usually adding an equal part of compound tincture of benzoin to that mixture.

Fume baths with rubdown; steam-cabinet treatments; massages; manipulative treatments; nose sprays and the already mentioned gargles with Glycothymoline and Listerine alternated; and a variety of cough syrups—all apparently were helpful in various circumstances to restore the body to a normal balance.

A most interesting suggestion was given to case 288-44: keep the body alkaline and eliminate the cold. Then Cayce said: "Instead of snuffing, BLOW! Instead of resentments, LOVE!"

Emphysema is a chronic, difficult-to-treat condition of the lungs in which much tissue has been destroyed and there is not much air exchange. It varies, of course, in severity. One of my favorite patients was afflicted with emphysema, and in October 1968 I started him using inhalations from a charred oak keg filled part way with apple brandy. He had a bit of trouble with his boss, who found his car—Jeff was an inspector in the field and drove a lot—smelling like a well-kept brewery, and insisted on a letter from me that said Jeff was smelling the fumes, not drinking the liquid. The fumes began having an effect, however, for it soon developed that it was not particularly curing my patient of emphysema, but it apparently was keeping him free of respiratory infections. Correspondence with the head of a national distillery confirmed that the fumes where the brandy was aged, in charred oak kegs, in fact kept employees free of any type of respiratory infections over a period of many, many years. Later, I had the opportunity to check up on Jeff and found that, in six years, since starting the inhalation, he had not been subject to a single infection in his respiratory tract. He did have flu once, but it was a generalized thing and did not affect his lungs or throat to any subjective degree.

Cayce suggested this particular type of inhalation therapy for nearly every case of tuberculosis. Here are some extracts that you might find interesting and stimulating:

> Prepare a charred oak keg, about a gallon-and-a-half to two-gallon keg. If a gallon and a half, put in same three-fourth gallon of Pure Apple Brandy.
>
> This keg should be so prepared that there would be two small openings in one end. One would act only as a vent when inhaling the fumes of the evaporated Brandy into the throat and lungs from the other opening, which would be prepared with a small tube—either of rubber or metal, or glass—that will not touch the brandy, but open into the vacuum above same, so that the fumes from the brandy may be inhaled two or three times a day. This should be kept where it will evaporate more quickly than ordinarily; not so much heat as to cause too great an evaporation, but where there is sufficient to create something more than the ordinary evaporation. Keep the vents tightly corked when not in use.
>
> 2978–1

> . . . Inhale these fumes 2 or 3 times a day. In the beginning do not inhale too much. Do inhale it, do not swallow it. While it will not hurt to swallow it, it is not as helpful to the body. The gas will not only act as an antiseptic, but will, with the properties that should be increased in the body, aid the change in the circulation, aiding these chemicals in their proper proportion to the body assimilation and the body activity, or the whole of the digestive forces, and eliminate the cause of infec-

tion in the lungs, proper, and we will find it will gradually heal those areas where at present there are openings, though not a great deal of live tubercle, but the adhesions as have been indicated are the more irritating for deep breathing.

5097—1

In discussing the problems found most commonly in tuberculosis, Cayce suggests that the basic findings here are a systemic alkalosis, or, more accurately, portions of the body are too alkaline, as well as a problem of assimilating foodstuffs into a circulatory system that lacks a proper activity in the pulmonary system itself . . . due mostly to the acid-alkaline imbalance.

Asthma, as seen in the Cayce readings, has its origin most commonly in the nervous system—pressures in the dorsal and sometimes the cervical ganglia or nerve cells. A variety of other causes either contribute to or actually cause the asthmatic condition, such as lesions that occur in the larynx and bronchial tree as the result of previous episodes of acute or chronic respiratory infection, or difficulties in gestation or at birth creating problems in the ganglia.

Therapy for the asthmatic patient (from the standpoint that these factors are causative) uses four concurrent approaches. First, the diet must be adjusted. In most individuals with asthma, the diet should be made more alkaline, for the body is usually overacid in its tissues. A diet, then, should be followed that includes a great deal of green vegetables and fruit, no fried foods, no pork, very little in the way of sweets or heavy starches, and fish, fowl, or lamb for the protein. Second, osteopathic adjustments, both specific and general, should be done in a cyclic fashion. Third, colonics should be given, where possible, weekly for two or three weeks, then perhaps once monthly; or enemas if colonics are not available.

Fourth, Cayce suggested Atomidine to be given in a series, to bring a balance to the glandular system, which he also saw as deficient. In case 1413, the patient was given one drop daily for five days in half a glass of water; then stopped for three days; then two drops daily for five days; then stopped again for three days; then back to the one drop daily for five days with a rest, and then two drops followed by the three-day rest, and then continued in this kind of cycle. Experience has taught us that the Atomidine is best placed in the glass first, then add the water so that the Atomidine is well mixed. The Atomidine, of course, is a prescription item and must be prescribed by a physician. We are not taught in medical school, however, to give drugs in a cyclic manner, so the method of administration suggested in the readings is probably a bit strange to most doctors.

Regular, daily bowel movements are important, sometimes a change in climate, sometimes an inhalant to be helpful in acute attacks. Much has already been written for physicians and for members of the A.R.E., and these should be sought out by anyone seriously interested in Cayce's suggestions about asthma.

In writing on the subject of respiratory allergy as it is discussed in the Cayce readings, Dr. Jim Kwako pointed out that the physical applications for correcting these problems focus on an inhalant, manipulation, and a controlled diet. The most common suggestion given to individuals with coryza, postnasal drainage, or sinusitis was an inhalant, and there were many formulations of what has come to be called the alcohol inhalant.

Cayce suggested that these are cleansers and are antiseptic for the mucous membranes of the respiratory tract. In one reading, he suggested that an eight-ounce bottle with a wide mouth be used, and a cork pierced with two glass tubes, one having a bulb at the end so that it may be placed to the nostril for inhaling the mixture. The instructions were to keep the bottle tightly corked until ready to use, then shake and inhale deeply into the lungs through each nostril, night and morning. In some instances, the directions were to inhale through the mouth, but many approaches were used—most of them to bring about the cleansing process by passing the fumes over the mucous membranes.

Listed below are three different compositions suggested in the readings, which show some of the variations that exist.

	(1)	(2)	(3)
Grain alcohol (at least 90 proof)	4 oz.	4 oz.	2 oz.
Oil of eucalyptus	20 minims	20 minims	30 minims
Rectified oil of turpentine	5 minims	5 minims	10 minims
Compound tincture of benzoin	15 minims	10 minims	20 minims
Oil of pine needles	10 minims		5 minims
Tolu, in solution	10 minims	30 minims	15 minims
Canadian balsam		5 minims	
Benzosol, saturated solution		5 minims	
Rectified creosote		3 minims	

Five or six drops of castor oil taken internally once a day is often useful to control and sometimes clear up the problem of allergies. We have used this therapy sometimes alone, and sometimes in conjunction with the other suggestions in this chapter.

Sinus problems often respond to Glycothymoline packs over the affected areas, and we also have used the therapy that Cayce suggested in the following quote:

Heat and combinations of the oils as indicated in mutton suet, spirits of turpentine, spirits of Camphor, and Compound Tincture of Benzoin. These remove congestion if heat is applied. For each carries with same activities upon the mucous membranes to aid in relieving, through penetration, healing and soothing.

341–43

It may be concluded that there are certain factors

that affect the alkalinity of the body tissues in the respiratory tract, that create an imbalance of the neurological control of that area, or that disturb the circulating blood to such an extent that changes come about in the cells of the lungs and other respiratory structures.

Bolting one's food, for instance, may set up problems, as may overheated rooms, overtiredness, loss of sleep, drafts, wet feet, or changes in temperature. Sometimes anger alone will do the job, and sometimes it is too much meat and starches. There are lots of causes. The correction usually involves more than one measure of therapy, but *always* involves an effort to establish a better total body balance.

Chapter Eighteen
THE DIGESTIVE ORGANS

In understanding what can easily be done to improve the total functioning of the digestive organs, we need to know that these organs involve the stomach, pancreas, liver, gallbladder, spleen, duodenum, jejunum, ileum, appendix, Peyer's patches, mesenteric lymph nodes, and the circulation of blood and lymph associated with all these structures. The emotions and the autonomic nerve supply to the organs of digestion also play a key part in the health or illness we experience.

When we look at the manner in which the ebb and flow of the sympathetic nerve supply to the digestive tract coordinates with the opposite activity of the parasympathetic to create the essential peristalsis or movement of food down the stomach and the intestinal tract, the process begins to become complicated. Then, when we consider the thymic (lymphatic or reticulo-endothelial) system, and its major role in assimilating food essentials, and the manner in which it also protects the body from foreign bodies, and the part it plays in maintaining the acid-alkaline balance, we see that eating our breakfast is not as simple as just putting food into our mouth, chewing it up, and swallowing it.

Further, we need to understand that the adrenal gland, frequently called the fight-flight gland, has an intimate relationship with the celiac (solar) plexus of nerves located in the central part of the abdominal cavity. The adrenal puts the entire body on the alert when danger appears or when a controversy arises at the dinner table, thereby working to shut down the activity of the digestive tract while sending blood out to the muscles so that they can be ready for action. The internal effect comes about partly through hormones but largely through the celiac plexus, the largest accumulation of nerve cells outside the head, which provides the entire area of digestion with sympathetic nerve fibers. If the energies of the body are not dissipated through action when they are aroused by the recognition of danger, problems gradually accumulate in the body, most commonly in the digestive tract.

So it is obvious that many forces are at work coordinating the pathways for the food that enters our mouth and arrives finally as molecular substances that can be gathered in by the living processes of cells throughout the body. Manipulating all these forces when they become deranged becomes an extremely difficult task. No wonder gastroenterology is a specialty in the field of medicine.

However, it is very important also to realize that the human body, when given a reasonable chance, will restore its balances to normal, and that we do not normally need to do a great deal of manipulation. This is the key to health in the digestive system as well as in other parts of the body.

We might ask, then, what do we need to do to aid those internal processes that lead to health?

1. Keep a proper diet.
2. Exercise regularly.
3. Reevaluate emotions and attitudes, and adopt new ones where a lack of constructive activity is indicated.

4. Correct inadequate eliminations through the bowel.
5. Correct acid-alkaline balance as nearly as possible.
6. Seek manipulative treatments as needed.
7. Study your dreams.
8. Do not fail to use prayer and meditation.
9. Add specifics where needed.

In caring for our bodies properly, we need to remember that our emotions are involved; that the outflow of nerves from the spinal cord, especially in the area of the fourth to the ninth dorsal vertebrae, are part of the picture; that the thymus system, the endocrine glands, and the parasympathetic and sympathetic nervous systems all play their roles; that the bloodstream and the lymphatic vessels bring life-giving substances and remove wastes from the tissues involved. Assimilation of foods and eliminatory activity go on all the time. How do we put all these things together? Sometimes we cannot, but it is always worthwhile to try, for we may be successful.

Preventive Measures

Edgar Cayce said many things while asleep that challenge one's imagination. For instance, we all have heard of ragweed, one of the most troublesome allergens. It is found everywhere, it seems, and the manufacturers of the desensitivity serums would be at a loss were it not for dust and ragweed. Cayce often referred to ragweed by its more romantic name, *Ambrosia* weed; and he saw in this remarkably bothersome plant a tremendously therapeutic ability.

Thanks to some careful research by Bob Clapp at the A.R.E. Headquarters in Virginia Beach, we find that this plant, when made into a tonic or a tea, can—according to Mr. Cayce—act to bring the entire intestinal tract into a better functioning condition. It can help the functioning of the liver, improve eliminations, and do all manner of remarkable things. Listen to this extract from the readings:

If there will be taken in the system, at regular intervals, those properties that are not habit forming, neither are they effective towards creating the condition where cathartics are necessary for the activities through the alimentary canal— whether related to the colon or the jejunum, or ileum—yet these will change the vibrations in such a manner as to keep clarified the assimilations, and aid the pancreas, the spleen, the liver, and the hepatic circulation, in keeping a normal equilibrium. The properties would be found in those of the Ambrosia weed made in this manner: To 6 oz. of distilled water, add 3 oz. of the *green* ragweed, or Ambrosia weed. Steep for sufficient period to reduce to half the quantity. Then strain, adding to this 2 oz. of simple syrup, with 1 oz. of grain alcohol. Shake the solution before the dose is taken. The dose would be half a teaspoon twice each day, when the period for taking has arisen—or take it about once a month, for three or four days. This will aid the digestive system, will aid the whole of the eliminating system.

454—1

Taking such a tea may be an excellent preventative of difficulties in the intestinal tract. Likewise, not eating too much, eating a reasonable alkaline-reacting diet, not arguing with your spouse while you eat, taking vitamins occasionally, making peace with yourself and others—all these are excellent preventatives for avoiding the situation where your body exclaims, "I just can't stomach that situation!" Or it might keep you from rebelling against the "gall" of your favorite enemy, who may in reality be yourself. Thus, we may prevent a stomach ulcer or a gall-bladder attack from materializing.

Practicing preventive measures, whether through the measures indicated above or through prayer and meditation, guidance through dreams, gaining insights through biofeedback or guided imagery, is preferable to correcting a medical problem once it has gained a foothold in the body.

The Stomach

Once a stomach ulcer has been treated successfully and then recurs, it is often very difficult to treat
the ulcer adequately. Perhaps this can be attributed
to fixed emotional and attitudinal responses, or deeply
set pathological changes. Yet, sometimes the response
to therapy is highly satisfactory, much to the joy of
the patient and the physician. Dr. S. J. Meda, one of
our referral medical doctors, reports that a thirty-
seven-year-old man, whom he had been treating for
a bleeding peptic ulcer (proven by X-ray), after a full
two and a half years of remission, experienced recurring symptoms intermittently with moderate severity for a period of four to five months. There were no
really significant physical findings—just the indigestion, discomfort, and "gas"; X-ray was not repeated.

The therapy in this case revolved around some of
the simplified suggestions in the Cayce material dealing with diet. Dr. Meda suggested a diet of fresh
vegetables, yogurt, bran, grapes, milk, and water in
abundance; and he had the patient avoid refined
sugar and flour, carbonated beverages, and fried
foods. Then the patient was instructed to drink saffron tea before meals. Patient response was highly
satisfactory, and the symptoms abated entirely after
four days, with no recurrence up to the time of Dr.
Meda's report, which was weeks after the initiation
of the diet. In a situation such as this, the Cayce
readings would also suggest that the basics of fish,
fowl, and lamb be added, while the restrictions indicated be continued.

Cleansing of the stomach can be brought about by
drinking quantities of pure water. However, Cayce
suggested elm water to several people who had considerable irritation; and he suggested that they drink
only this as water intake. Elm water is prepared by
putting a pinch of powdered elm in a cup of water
that has had an ice cube added. After allowing the
mixture to steep or soak for three minutes, drink it
cool. Elm water apparently counteracts the acidity
present.

Saffron tea, made with yellow or American saffron, was also suggested frequently in the readings to "coat the whole of the stomach proper." This tea should be taken just prior to each meal and can be made by adding three teaspoons of saffron to sixteen ounces of hot water and letting it steep for one-half to three-quarters of an hour. However, if a meal consists entirely of raw vegetables, it is not necessary to take any saffron beforehand. On occasion, Cayce suggested a teaspoon of Milk of Magnesia to be taken after each meal—the purpose being to cleanse and quiet the condition of the stomach.

To one enquiring individual (389-9), a fifty-nine-year-old man who had previously received other direction from Cayce, several suggestions were made to improve assimilation. First, he was given instructions regarding diet, similar to those that have already been given. Second, Cayce suggested some regular massage, and specifically that the man have an electrical vibrator massage treatment regularly, using the vibrator alongside the entire spine and down the extremities. Finally, he was told to take a teaspoon of Bisodol a half-hour after the heavy meal of the day.

A woman (2452–1), who had been undergoing considerable emotional strain, was having digestive difficulties. To her Cayce suggested the following regimen: 6 drops of Elixir of Lactated Pepsin in water taken after the heavy meal of the day for two days; on the third day, 10 drops of the same material in ⅔ glass of water and adding ½ teaspoon of Milk of Bismuth; then, on the fourth day, she was instructed to take a colonic. She was also advised to have the vibratory massage treatments.

For a man (19–3) who was experiencing hyperacidity of the stomach, a different course of therapy was suggested. Alkaline substances such as Glycothymoline or Lavoris were used as a gargle, swallowing a few drops of the material left in the mouth; saffron and camomile teas were also suggested, made up half and half, and allowed to steep for thirty minutes and taken several times one day. Then, on the next day, a teaspoon of Milk of Magnesia and a teaspoon of Milk of Bismuth were to be taken. This routine was to be followed, on alternating days, and on the third day a massage could be given.

The Gallbladder

While overacidity and ulceration of the stomach is the most common problem in the intestinal organs of digestion and assimilation, gallbladder trouble probably runs a close second. Cholecystitis (inflammation of the gallbladder) and cholelithiasis (formation of stones in the gallbladder) are felt by many to be related chronologically: the inflammation comes first, followed by the development of stones. Even while this theory is debated, the real reason behind the development of any pathology of the gallbladder remains to some extent obscure. Emotions certainly play a large part, perhaps creating the structure within which the real problems can develop.

According to a report to the British Medical Association by Dr. K. W. Heaton (University of Bristol), gallstones and the underlying gallbladder disease that must be present for the stones to be formed are the product of civilization and its refinements. The real culprits, he points out, are the refined carbohydrates that, when ingested regularly, cause more weight gain and are sweeter and easier to digest, but have less of the essential fiber and are less bulky, less chewy, and less satisfying in the long run. Thus, for the sake of the gallbladder, it remains the responsibility of each individual to fashion a diet for his or her own consumption out of foods that are not refined. The fiber present in the unrefined products sold at the corner supermarket is a great preventive of intestinal cancer.

In the Edgar Cayce readings there were consistent suggestions relative to diet for those individuals who had gallbladder disease:

The general diet would be:

Mornings—stewed fruits, with rice cakes, or whole wheat bran cakes, or coarse ground meal cakes, see? A little tea or coffee, not too strong.

Noon—as many of the green vegetables as may be
well made into a salad which may be eaten with
dressing of the oil base; that is, whether the French
dressing or mayonnaise—either would be well. At
this period it would be well that some milk be
taken, of one nature or another, preferably butter-
milk, or that which has been treated with that
that produces the proper fermentation.

Evenings—small quantities of meat, but these
should only be those that do not carry fats.

356–1

In the matter of the diet, keep away from fried
foods. Do increase the amount of raw foods; that
is, lettuce, celery, carrots, radishes, all of those
that are taken as salads—with mayonnaise at times
and at others have these prepared with gelatin.

5024–1

In the Cayce material, most often the therapy for
stones in the gallbladder is a cautious one. The diet
is corrected first, then an individual is often given
manipulative treatments, and castor oil packs are
administered to the abdomen for several consecutive
days. Olive oil is then administered by mouth. The
amount varies according to what the individual is
able to take without upsetting his stomach. The
amount can vary from a teaspoon to half a cup or
more. But caution is the word. And the procedures
are repeated until relief is obtained. Over the years,
we have received reports that when such recommendations are followed, results are forthcoming and
the stones are excreted through the bile and common duct into the intestinal tract.

We need to understand the perspective that Cayce
used in approaching a definition of what he "saw"
in the person for whom he was giving a reading.
They were always seen as individuals, as entities
with creative ability who had in reality created the
disease process found existing in the body. Thus,
cholelithiasis is not in reality an entity in itself, and
should not be treated as such; rather, each person,
through a series of circumstances, builds the poten-

tial for stones within his or her own body; and the
result produces large stones in one person, grape-
sized ones in another, and gravel-sized in a third.
Because the etiology or origin of the disease is
different in each person, Cayce saw fit to individualize
the therapy program suggested. This doesn't mean
that a standard therapy program is not a good thing,
but rather that each person should be looked at
individually, and the physician or therapist should
give some consideration to the nature of this individ-
uality. Thus, the only way for one person may be
surgery to have the stones removed, while another
might easily pass the stones if conditions and therapy are right.

In reading 5060–1, Cayce saw sediment in the
gallbladder. His treatment plan was simple: use a
castor oil pack over the abdomen for five days in a
row, then start taking olive oil by mouth, one teaspoon every four hours for five days. A different
program of therapy was designed for the man who
carried the reading number 2278–1. He was told
also to take castor oil packs daily for five days, but
while doing these, he should lie on his right side
with a pillow under the gallbladder area, so that
the gallbladder would drain. Then, after the series
of packs, he was to take two teaspoons of olive
oil. A third program was given for case 1857–1.
He was told to take several weeks of therapy, using
the castor oil packs three consecutive days each
week, followed by two teaspoons of olive oil each
time.

Frequently, in other readings, Cayce would suggest larger or smaller amounts of olive oil. He nearly
always recommended the use of castor oil packs.
Diet was consistently a part of therapy. Sometimes
he would suggest massage over the abdomen, sometimes colonics or osteopathy, and sometimes an electric vibrator to be used over the spine.

Here is a story about the gallbladder and its tra-
vails from a woman who had only recently become a
member of the A.R.E. She wrote me this letter about
her experience, which became for her a change in
consciousness:

I had suffered from abdominal pains for fifteen or more years but had considered them merely "gas pains." Having a history of ulcers and not being one to run to a doctor for every little pain, I suffered in silence. I carried baking soda with me always.

However, last fall, after returning from a stay at A.R.E., of which I had only recently become a member, I found my personal life in a very unsettled state. The pains, which had usually come and gone in an erratic way, were now always with me! Within an hour after eating, especially in the evening, I would be doubled up with pain and spend hours every night walking up and down the patio, trying to obtain relief, until finally I was able to sleep from sheer exhaustion!

I had naturally turned to God in my misery. However, the turmoil in my private life seemed to be in the way of my usual rapport. I struggled constantly with my hate, fear, doubt, and dissolution!

One night I sat alone around two in the morning. I had been going through my Edgar Cayce and A.R.E. books, hoping to find an answer, a treatment to try. Before me were the "Palma Christi" and the A.R.E. #1 Black Book. I opened the Black Book at random—I did not look down at it immediately, but sat staring into space. When I finally looked down at the book open before me— there at the top of the right-hand page in heavy black print were two words—GALL BLADDER. I was stunned. I read the article immediately—every word was imprinted on my mind—a great feeling of relief came over me. I knew, I knew!

Just simple castor oil treatments with a heating pad over the abdomen and well up over the gallbladder in a series of three times on and three times off, with the taking of pure olive oil on alternate days. Two in the morning was no time to start castor oil treatments, so I went to bed knowing that at last my search had been answered.

The next evening, choosing the hour of nine, I started the treatments. Relief was apparent at once!

After two series as recommended, the pains were completely gone. I have kept the treatments up over a period of three months and then off for several months and the pain has never returned! I can eat almost anything I please with no bad aftereffects.

Now comes the odd part!

I had never discussed my experience with anyone, but a friend, complaining about her stomach troubles, inquired what I had done for mine. I went looking for the article and I have searched both the Black Book and the "Palma Christi" numerous times, but as I saw it that night, it is not there!

The Liver

The gallbladder is, in a sense, just a storage place for bile that is produced by the liver, so it may be called upon to produce that bile and discharge it into the duodenum when it is needed. The liver tucks the gallbladder up underneath its belly and shelters it, making it a bit difficult for the surgeon when he is given the task of removing the gallbladder. But the liver is the big organ and certainly one of the most important in the entire human body. Its functions are multitudinous—it has been called the "great detoxifier" and it produces more lymph than any other portion of the body. Its bile aids both in elimination of substances and in digestion. It is important in most of our life-support systems.

Hepatitis is the most evident problem afflicting the liver. Infectious hepatitis regularly responds well to the use of castor oil packs and a strong, supportive dietary regimen. One of the most pleasing responses occurred in the case of a fifty-nine-year-old man who developed hepatitis in the guise of an apparent intestinal flu. On his second visit to the Clinic, it became obvious that our original diagnosis was incorrect, and the infectious hepatitis became obvious, supported by laboratory findings. He had already started castor oil packs to his abdomen on our recommendation because of the distension and dis-

comfort of the abdomen, which had brought him
into the Clinic in the first place. Thus, on his second visit, in spite of his jaundiced (yellowed) appearance, he was feeling somewhat better. His liver was
enlarged two to three finger-breadths down from the
rib margin. His diet was mostly clear liquids and a
basically light diet with very little starch or protein.
He improved daily, and on the fifth day he was started
on a blender mix that was prepared from water,
unsweetened frozen fruit, protein powder, and yeast
powder. Fish was added to his diet and he reported
clinical improvement daily. He was ambulatory but
was encouraged to rest a lot. His laboratory findings
improved from a high on the second day to a normal-
ization of all reports on the twenty-eighth day. The
SGPT count was the last to return to normal, moving from a high of 755 on the first test to 40 on the
last. The jaundice disappeared rapidly, and the total
bilirubin in the blood returned to normal on the
fifteenth day. On the nineteenth day, the patient
was released to return to work, feeling normal in all
respects. The diet remained a light one, with fish,
fowl, and lamb as the only proteins, and with vegetables and fruits high on the list of foods to be taken.
The blender mix was continued along with the diet
through the next two months. The castor oil packs
were continued daily for three weeks, then used just
three days a week thereafter for three months.

One of our nurses at the Clinic was able to finish
nurse's training because she followed a regimen like
the one given above during a period of short vaca-
tion and sick-time after she made her own diagnosis.
Not letting her school know the details, she used
castor oil packs, diet, and some meditation experiences that gave her new insights on herself and
facilitated the complete clearing of the symptoms
and the abnormal findings. Had she missed more
school, she would not have been allowed to go back,
so it was a critical time for her.

The illnesses associated with the liver, the gallbladder, and the stomach constitute the majority of
difficulties experienced in the upper intestinal tract.
There are also splenic and pancreatic malfunctions.

The most common pancreatic disturbance is caused by a diminished function of the islets of Langerhans in the pancreas. It is a condition we call diabetes, or an excess of sugar in the blood.

Acid-Alkaline Balance

In my experience, nearly all the functions of the digestive organs and their nerve and vascular supply can be improved by paying attention to and working to correct the acid-alkaline balance. It is never fully informational to test the saliva or the urine for the pH, since there is a constant pH in the bloodstream, and the cells of the body can become slightly too acid or too alkaline. It is in the functioning cells of any organ, gland, or system that influences of a detrimental nature can bring about a disease of the body.

It is difficult to determine simply whether a physical body is too acid or too alkaline. Cayce suggested that the serious, chronic illnesses like rheumatoid arthritis and scleroderma were overalkaline, this being a much more difficult condition to correct. And he suggested also that if a body were to stay slightly alkaline, which is normal, that body would never catch a cold. Apparently, body defenses are dropped somewhat when the body gets to be even slightly acid.

There are foods—starches, sweets, and meats, primarily—that are acid reacting in their nature. There are others that are more neutral—like milk, for instance. And there are others that react in the body to create an alkaline state—fruits and vegetables, mainly. What this means is that a diet, if followed strictly, can bring about a more alkaline state in the body if it is fashioned mostly of alkaline-reacting foodstuffs. The opposite, of course, is also true. This helps in understanding what happens to the body when certain dietary habits are followed. Cayce pointed out that sweets, chocolate, and starches were the prime causative agents of skin problems such as acne and psoriasis. Perhaps these problems are the skin's response to an overload of nonuseful substances in the bloodstream that need to be eliminated.

There are also activities that we take part in as human beings that make the body cells more acid or more alkaline. Exercise makes for a slight alkalinity. A sedentary job, thinking, working with the mind and not the body, fussing, arguing, worrying—all these make for greater acidity. The nervous system activity associated with exercise is sympathetic, associated with adrenal output, and it creates a slight alkalinity. On the other hand, the parasympathetic nervous system is active during worry, thinking, sitting, arguing, fussing, etc. It is the function of the vagus nerve (the cervical parasympathetic) to cause acid to be secreted into the stomach as a part of the digestive process. The adrenal (sympathetic), on the other hand, through its function in exercise, causes the stomach activity to shut down and causes a stoppage of the acid flow into the stomach.

For purposes of simplicity—not necessarily for accuracy—we might look at things as if worry and thinking and tension activate the parasympathetic nervous system, which uses up the alkalinity in the body and produces acid. Exercise does the opposite for the sympathetic—it uses up the acid and produces alkalinity. Generally, it is true that physically hard-working people are not ulcer people. Those who have jobs that require little activity of the physical body are more subject to ulcers. The stress and worry and frustration that also cause ulcers can be present in either group, so tension-caused overacidity is a problem common to all groups of people.

To bring correction means many things. It can be done simply by using diet or exercise additions such as were discussed earlier to make the body more alkaline and to improve eliminations—for "drosses" in the bloodstream cause a disruption of the lymph flow, which, incidentally, is normally alkaline. When the lymph becomes slightly acid, the lymphocytes do not function well. And the resistance to disease is lowered, for the lymphocytes are the primary defenders in the bloodstream. Cayce called them the "warriors."

Correction of the acid-alkaline balance may necessitate a change in lifestyle. It may mean adopting a new way of looking at things, so that contentment can come instead of frustration. There are always at least two ways of looking at things. It may require the development of a changed attitude. "First, change your attitude toward the mental and spiritual. Then do these things." This was the way Edgar Cayce often expressed the underlying principle—an essential principle to remember as well as to practice.

Chapter Nineteen
LOWER BOWEL DIFFICULTIES

The lower bowel and its associated structures are intimately related to the organs of digestion, for without a balance being achieved between assimilation and elimination, health in the lower bowel cannot long exist. Among the more common ailments we will consider in this chapter are constipation and its opposite, diarrhea. Colitis can be a more serious situation involving either inadequate or, more frequently, excessive bowel movements. Diverticulitis, inflammation of the sacs branching out from the intestines, is a problem for many people. Finally, there are hemorrhoids, which occur almost as frequently as constipation and often appear to be a result of this constipation.

Since the large lower bowel, in its entirety, is the only major structure involved in this discussion, there are not too many functions to concern ourselves with: the cells of the bowel itself, the lymph and blood supply, and the autonomic nerve fibers directing the activities of the bowel throughout its course. Despite its apparent simplicity, however, and perhaps because of its extreme importance to the total body function, problems in the lower bowel exist more frequently than in any other part of the body. People are either chronically constipated or acutely troubled. Diarrhea or hemorrhoids are a frequent concern, and a psychological "fixation" on the lower bowel and its functions is not uncommon. Psychologists recognize that individuals who do not express their thoughts, feelings, and emotions commonly complain of constipation. They hold things in physically, showing to the world, in a sense, the message that they are unable to express verbally.

While my patients and my correspondents are not as thrilled at correcting constipation as they are at using an inhalant to clear up a cold, it is undoubtedly more important, for the body needs to eliminate those substances that we consider waste products. If we do not, we die; it is that important. Furthermore, if the function of that portion of the body becomes chronically disturbed, the lower bowel symptoms usually manifest early on, but the rest of the body becomes ill eventually. Either the job of eliminating gets transferred to another one of the eliminatory organs and that function reaches overload and breaks down, or the accumulation of toxins and byproducts of metabolism destructively influences the function of digestion or the vascular system. A balance of health means that both assimilation and elimination must work normally. There is no way to avoid this fact.

Diverticulitis

Upgrading the lower bowel in its function means normalizing the peristalsis (wavelike muscular contractions) and the neurological supply to the muscles of the rectum. It means bringing adequate blood supply to the bowel walls; bringing back to normal the lymphatic flow through the lymphatic vessels and nodes of the bowel and the mesentery, the membranous folds connecting the intestines to the rear abdominal walls; and cleansing the cells and giving them the stimulus to respond in a normal fashion. These goals are seldom easy to reach, mainly because the mind and emotions are so closely interrelated to bodily function, and it is always difficult to change one's attitudes. After all, we have held them close to us for a long time; somtimes, however, very simple procedures at the physical level will bring about changes in consciousness that are needed, and a tremendous response results.

One of life's great privileges for me has been the opportunity to visit on several occasions with Sarah Hesson, Edgar Cayce's only living sister. She wrote us recently and told us of her use of castor oil packs:

> I'm writing you to tell you of my recent experience with castor oil packs (however, I'm completely sold on them because I've always had such wonderful benefits from them).
>
> When I was in the hospital a year ago, and had so many X-rays, Dr. Gupton reported to me, besides a couple of broken bones, I had "diverticulitis," which would have to be reckoned with. Well, last week, in the evening, a pain hit me in the colon—quite severe, though it would come and go. I went to bed and fell asleep without doing anything to relieve it—but was awakened in the early morning hours with the same severe pain—so I got up and fixed a castor oil pack, put it on, and went back to bed. After having it on for several hours, I would feel the *severeness* of the pain subsiding, and by noon it was entirely gone and has not returned. However, for three successive nights I repeated the packs and have been more careful with my diet. I thought it was really miraculous.

Our experience has taught us that most problems associated with diverticulosis can be controlled by using the castor oil packs regularly, and gradually bringing the diet around to contain more of the roughage that is usually denied the patient who has this problem. Diverticulitis (the inflammation), and the condition itself, without the irritation—diverticulosis—is most frequently associated with constipation. I have never seen X-ray evidence of diverticuli or sacs actually disappearing once they have appeared on the scene, but I am convinced that it can happen. The need is to make the permanent changes in function, thought, emotion, and lifestyle that brought the condition into being in the first place. If a start is made in that direction, and the physical applications are followed through, the change in the bowel may then come about.

Constipation

Most often, constipation has its origin in an acidity created by the assimilating system of the body. As we discussed earlier, the Edgar Cayce readings indicate that stress, tension states, arguments, disagreements, anger, and other negative manifestations of the adrenal gland activity bring such acidity into being in the stomach-duodenal area.

With excess acid present in the stomach, our lymphatic function decreases, creating an inactivity of the liver; this leads to a declining production of enzymes and a subsequent decrease in proper digestion and assimilation. This, in turn, cuts down markedly on the forces available for producing normal eliminations. Thus, various foods that at other times are acceptable to the body become poisons, and the system becomes overloaded with "used and refused forces": the end products of metabolism, the foods that are refused by the body, the substances produced by improper metabolism, and the intestinal wastes that are being reabsorbed through the lower intestinal walls. After this occurs, there arises a condition that might be described as an intestinal indigestion that causes a packing of fecal material in the large bowel. This condition is what we know as constipation.

It must be recognized that constipation occurs as a result of various types of diseases, but the development as described above is probably the most common. Associated with constipation nearly always, and sometimes acting as a cause, are varying pressures and minor dislocations of the cervical, dorsal, and lumbar regions. An improper diet, such as an acid-reacting meat-and-potatoes diet, kept up as a regular procedure, is also a major factor.

The consequences of constipation are consistently

underrated, quite possibly because they are not understood. When the toxins or poisons are reabsorbed into the cirulation, the liver loses even more its ability to excrete as well as to secrete those substances that it should. The kidneys usually respond to this declining activity of the liver by becoming overtaxed in their own function of eliminating substances from the body; then there appear symptoms of dysuria (painful or difficult urination) associated with inflammation of the kidney, the bladder, and the tubes associated with the related renal system. The skin and lungs—our other two organs of elimination—are then called upon to exercise their functions more vigorously in order to keep the body in a reasonable general balance. Halitosis, respiratory ailments, or various skin disturbances may occur initially; but when the situation advances and becomes more severe, serious illnesses in these two systems may come about.

How did Cayce approach such a problem? With each person he gave a program that was just a little bit different. However, I think you will find this one interesting and fairly representative. He was discussing the nervous system.

... Here we find there has been a great deal of taxation in the system of WORRYING over things that are on the mind of the entity—many of which have never happened, many may never happen, but these become to the body at times just as disturbing as if they were a part of the experience.

This is the inclination that brings to the system those depressions through the nerve forces of the body.

Then, with those conditions where there has been the slowing up of the activity, there needs to be better coordination between the cerebrospinal and the sympathetic system,—especially in the areas of the 9th dorsal; relaxing those throughout the upper portion of the dorsal and lower cervical, and some corrections in the sacral and lumbar areas. These should be relaxed opposite one from

another,—that is, first those in the areas from
the 9th dorsal to the cervicals, then those in the
lumbar and sacral areas, and lastly the coordination of the 9th dorsal with both the cervical AND
the upper dorsal areas. These treatments would
be given twice a week.

Also we would begin as soon as practical,—tomorrow or the day after, you see,—and have a high
colonic irrigation. Then in about ten days have
another. Then in two weeks have another. Then
perhaps it would be a month before the next would
be given. The same one who gives the osteopathic
manipulations should give the colonics, see?

The evening BEFORE the colonic irrigations are
to be given the next day, you see, we would apply
the hot Castor Oil Packs over the area of the liver
AND the caecum,—that is, along the right side.
Have at least three thicknesses of flannel, making
the heavy Castor Oil Packs, and apply direct to
the body for at least two or three hours. A hot pad
may be put over same to hold the heat in same,
—not enough to be over irritating, but enough to
relax the system so that the colonic irrigations
will reduce—gradually—this plethoric condition,
—that causes pressures through the nerve forces
upon the gall duct and the liver area. These Packs
would be applied ONLY at the period when the
high colonic irrigations are to be given the next
day, see?

Do not take a great deal of medicinal properties.
Use laxatives, to be sure, when necessary; but for
THIS body we would advise taking a fruit salts
laxative. The Eno Salts would be very well, and is
a fruit salts.

In the matter of the diet—keep to a great deal of
the fruit juices and a great deal of the raw foods
taken especially at one meal during the day;
whether evening, noon or just which meal depends upon the body. No fried foods at ALL, EVER!
The green or fresh vegetables are very well. . . .

                                              1930–1

In another instance, where the kidneys and the stomach had already been affected by the reabsorption of bodily wastes, he suggested the Milk of Bismuth and Elixir of Lactated Pepsin and also osteopathic treatments, but this was his advice relative to the constipation:

> We would, however, be more mindful as to the diet; and as the seasons change it will be well that there be more of the vegetables, and at least one or two vegetables or a combination of vegetables taken raw (but fresh).
>
> The Eno Salt—a teaspoonful taken each morning before any meal for five days, then left off for a week and then begun again, and this procedure repeated for three to four periods or rounds—would aid in cleansing the system, and be a mild activity upon the kidneys in alleviating the drosses from the system.
>
> 1191–3

A nineteen-year-old boy had developed cellulitis, or inflammation of the tissue just below the skin. Cayce gave suggestions for local applications, but also indicated the need of a bodily cleansing through the bowels: "As an eliminant, we would give Castor Oil; followed in forty-eight hours afterwards with broken doses of Fletcher's Castoria."   670–3

I think that in all instances where there is a severe inflammation and the body is throwing off toxins and the residue of dead cells into the circulation, elimination must be increased and aided if the body is going to function adequately. This is not recognized by most physicians—simply because the stress in medical schools is not toward an applied physiology of function, but toward therapy of diseases.

For children, Cayce usually suggested Castoria. A six-year-old boy had been having intermittent fevers, and "congestions through the alimentary canal." For him, Cayce made the following recommendations:

There have been some distresses produced in the caecum and the liver area, as we find, by adhesions.

We would apply first the Castor Oil packs over the caecum and the lacteal duct area, as hot as the body may stand same; first, to relax the body, you see.

Then, after the packs have been kept for three to four hours (changing them, of course, as they cool), we would then begin giving the broken doses of Fletcher's Castoria for the removal of the fecal forces through the system that make for poisonings. This should be given in broken doses; that is, half a teaspoonful every half hour until there are two or three full and complete movements through the alimentary canal from same.

927–1

It becomes evident from searching the readings that one major means of cleansing the body is through aiding the alimentary canal to avoid what often occurs in a state of illness—that is, the reabsorption into the bloodstream of products of body life activities. These products need to be eliminated *from* the bloodstream. Unless normal bowel activity is maintained, the effects on the rest of the body can be far-reaching and sometimes quite serious.

Hemorrhoids

One of the more troublesome complications or results of constipation is the vascular change that we call hemorrhoids, which comes about at the anal opening. The condition is just a breakdown of the integrity of the veins in the anal area. Due to straining, the venous walls distend, and gradually the problem comes into being. Hemorrhoids are difficult to treat successfully, if you wish to obtain a medical rather than a surgical solution to the problem. Most of the patients I have treated for this condition are not willing to go through the steps that Cayce recommended. It is difficult for all of us to change habits in a consistent, life-altering manner when we are given a problem such as hemorrhoids—a problem that we do not like to talk about and that does not seem so serious. However, there are problems behind such problems, and we must eventually come face to face with ourselves. Here is what Cayce had to say to a sixty-two-year-old woman suffering from hemorroids

> A-2: Change the conditions in the body. Prepare a combination of oils to be injected. This may cause a bit of irritation but using this regularly, about once every ten days, we may eliminate these conditions entirely. Put two drops of carbolic acid in one once of glycerine and beat together very thoroughly, then add two ounces of Usoline. Stir, mix or shake this very thoroughly, and then use a baby syringe for injecting into the rectum—this quantity should be sufficient for at least two or three injections. This will remove the tensions there. But it is more important to stir the circulation and the eliminations, and to remove the toxic forces in the manners indicated. This will eliminate the soreness in the duodenum, through the alimentary canal and relieve the tension on the heart, the liver and kidneys. And the throat should clear up in the first series of applications to the gall duct and caecum area.

> 3550—1

The "applications" referred to in this reading had to do with abdominal castor oil packs. He had also suggested colonics, fume baths with witch hazel, general full-body massages, and certain dietary precautions. These suggestions, as usual, were aimed at specific conditions in the body where needed, but seemed more importantly directed at balancing the energies and the nervous systems and circulation of the entire body. Again, it is the story of the whole body that gets told when Cayce gives a reading—and it should be the whole body that we work with and try to bring back to wholeness.

A common Cayce recommendation for relief of hemorrhoids is an exercise of stretching up high with both arms, holding the hip muscles tight and then bending forward and regularly repeating this several times daily. One stands on his toes during this experience, which makes it more difficult, and does the bending six times each period.

Colitis

Colitis, an inflammation of the colon, is frequently a rather serious disease. It may occur in the very young or in the adult, and it may be spastic or mucous colitis. Problems occur here, as in constipation (although with different results), because the problem always occurs in conjunction with lymphatic disturbances. The lacteal ducts throughout the intestinal tract, the lymphatic vessels, the lymph nodes, and the Peyer's patches are all involved in a sometimes inflammatory condition. Because of the inflammation in the walls of the intestine, the lymph fluid itself often becomes toxic to the entire body and particularly to the liver. Because of the toxic effect on the Peyer's patches and the lacteal ducts, both of which are closely related to the assimilatory process, the food that is ingested can no longer be assimilated properly and thereby made ready to participate in the rebuilding of body tissues.

A one-month-old child was given a reading (2892) because of his acute colitis. The response was immediate and dramatic when he was placed on a regimen of drastic underfeeding; two drops of Glycothymoline three times a day; daily enemas with some Glycothymoline in the enema water (sometimes olive oil was used first as an enema); Glycothymoline packs across the abdomen, put on as hot as could be stood and left on until cool (fifteen to twenty minutes) two or three times daily; one or two drops of Castoria each hour until movement is obtained every two or three days; and yellow saffron tea sipped in minute quantities during the day, made up fresh daily. In just a few hours the baby had recovered, but the therapy continued until the body was made a bit more normal. This always seems to be a rule that

one should follow: don't just get rid of the symptoms—
instead, work to return the body to a normal condition.

In all these instances, Cayce did not remind those
who were searching that they should have a better
attitude toward spiritual things, that they should be
meditating or praying daily, or that all the applications should be applied in an attitude that would
bring wholeness through the activity of the Spirit
working in the very tissues of the body. He apparently followed his own recommendation to another
person: "If you have a castor oil consciousness, use
castor oil." When people asked for help, it was given
in the way that they could understand. If they followed instructions closely and patiently, persistently
and consistently, positive results would come about.
Cayce once said that there was as much of God in a
teaspoon of castor oil as there was in a prayer.

In working with colitis in the adult, the story is a
bit different. The diet he suggested to one person
was:

> Keep away from meats. Only fish or fowl may be
> taken, and these never fried. NO FRIED FOODS
> OF ANY KIND. Take rather the body-building and
> strength-giving foods—especially a great deal of
> fruits, fruit-juices—including citrus fruit juices,
> of course. Combine a little lemon with the orange
> juice. Plenty of prunes, prune whip. Plenty of pine-
> apple and the like. All of these would be the
> principals, though not all of the diet. Refrain from
> a great deal of pastries. Malted milks and those of
> such natures may be in the diet. Not too much of
> candies or sweets, though occasionally milk in
> chocolate or cocoa or the like may be taken.
>
> 2085–1

Restoring the lymphatics back to normal involves
six steps, according to the Cayce readings:

1. Rest.
2. Eliminate the inflammatory process.
3. Balance the acid-alkaline ratio in the body by
   soothing the activity of the lymphatics.

4. Cleanse the lymphatics.
5. Balance the eliminations and the liver function.
6. Coordinate the nervous-system activity.

Specifics that Cayce recommended were Glyco-thymoline packs to the abdomen; Concord grapes, crushed, applied over the abdomen for one and a half to four hours; mild exercise in the open air; massage with camphorated oil to the abdomen and to the spine; osteopathic treatments; and simply more rest. There is also a fusion of wild ginseng available, which is one of the prime therapies used for colitis.

Diarrhea

King Tut's Curse is what diarrhea is called when a tourist visits Egypt and acquires this disorder. Here in Arizona, we call it Montezuma's Curse. In the Center for Disease Control in Atlanta, the syndrome is aptly called *tourista,* and they now have a cure for it that has had clinical trials among the Apache Indian children and the children of Bangladesh ref-uge camps—areas where diarrhea has been a severe problem. The cure sounds like it was derived from the ancients and their wisdom, but the director of the study, Dr. Eugene J. Gangarosa, did not divulge the source of the cure. The procedure is simple:

Use two drinking glasses. Into the first, pour eight ounces of fruit juice. Add a half teaspoonful of honey or corn syrup and a pinch of salt. Into the second glass, pour eight ounces of boiled or car-bonated water, adding one-fourth teaspoonful of baking soda.

To use the remedy, one should take a swallow from one glass, followed by a swallow from the other, alternating until the two glasses are empty.

In the August 20, 1977, issue of the *Arizona Republic,* Julian DeVries, medical editor, quotes Gangarosa as explaining that the diarrhea experi-

enced by the tourists is nature's way of flushing out
poisonous substances. "Drugs that halt the process,"
he said, "are thwarting nature." It sounds like efforts to treat the patient instead of "the disease"
have at last invaded one of the strongholds of science.

Cayce saw the need for a balance in the intestinal
tract as highly important. At times he suggested
that diarrhea came about because of the lack of
proper assimilation of foods; and, at other times,
because of the introduction of toxic substances, such
as might be found in foods or drinks that are not
normal to the individual. He suggested the therapy
of castor oil packs to the abdomen, along with a
glass of water into which had been added a teaspoon
of Milk of Bismuth and ten drops of Elixir of Lactated Pepsin—the water then to be well mixed and
taken slowly. At times, osteopathic manipulations
were suggested. In an infant who had diarrhea, he
gave the following suggestion:

> Give small doses—a few drops of Glycothymoline,
> in almost all the water taken. This as an intesti-
> nal antiseptic will keep down inflammation in
> colon.
>
>   2289–6

In both the Cayce suggestions and the treatment
regimen developed by the Center for Disease Control
in Atlanta, diet is central. The C.D.C. has kept its
patients on a very limited diet: additional carbonated beverages, boiled water or tea, no solid foods or
milk. The Cayce material likewise recommends no
solid foods at first, then gradually switching to a
diet that eliminates starches for the most part. This
is what we call an alkaline-reacting diet, which builds
resistance to such intestinal upsets; and I'm sure
that Cayce had in mind the Peyer's patches when he
made such suggestions, for these patches—in the
context of the readings—are very important areas of
healing, assimilation, and control of the acid-base
balance of the body.

Perhaps the most important thing to remember
about the lower bowel and its care is the fact that all

things, mechanical and living, seem to perform their more normal function while clean. The human body certainly needs cleanliness, both in the body and in the mind—and we can make our state of being more what it should be by keeping the function of the lower bowel up to par, thereby cleansing the body in many ways.

Chapter Twenty
THE BLADDER AND KIDNEYS

The urinary tract as a unit comprises one of four systems of elimination in the human body—the other three being: the liver and intestines, the lungs, and the skin. It is probably a fact that the kidneys and bladder will not malfunction if the other eliminatory organs are kept in proper balance. Trouble really begins when other parts of the body begin to influence the function of the kidneys and the bladder. At that point, disease really has its onset.

A survey of the Cayce readings reveals that most cases of cystitis, or inflammation of the urinary bladder, for instance, are associated with disease states in other parts of the body. In very few instances was cystitis the only condition, or even the major condition, for which a reading was given. This points us toward the need to maintain good general body health in preventing cystitis.

It is interesting that Cayce sees the hepatic or liver-related circulation as involving the kidneys as well; and he apparently includes the portal vein circulation and the arterial supply to the liver as the remainder of the hepatic circulation. The portal circulation is the venous flow from the organs of digestion that goes directly to the liver before entering the venous system and returning to the heart. Cayce described it in this way:

As an organ (for the more perfect understanding of the body, for this may be disputed by some), the liver and the kidneys form the hepatic circulation. The blood supply of the whole body goes through the liver twice, even to once through the heart.

1140-2

In other instances, Cayce saw disturbance to the hepatic circulation coming from a variety of functional disturbances, few of which might be given a proper name in our present scheme of medical nomenclature—e.g., prolapsed descending colon, disturbances in the red cell element of the blood, cerebrospinal lesions, torpid liver, etc. And most of these problems create a tendency to overacidity and subsequent irritation or inflammation of the bladder or other portions of the system. If measures can be taken early in this process, health is much more easily restored and crisis medicine need not be required—and that is the ideal. Unfortunately, the soul's need for learning often brings about the full-blown disease, and it must be cared for creatively or allowed to take its course.

The key to prevention of renal or kidney tract problems is found in maintaining an alkaline balance in the body tissues and in keeping a general state of health for the whole body. In other words, have you started a good diet, an exercise program, regular prayer and meditation, an upgrading of your emotions and attitudes? Do you study your dreams for guidance? Have you worked with your mind in visual imagery, autogenic exercises, or in providing an intake of constructive mind food through your reading or viewing? When these things are done, very little trouble will usually be found in this area of the eliminatory organs. When trouble does occur, however, there are other measures that might be taken to help create health once again:

1. Continue the *preventive efforts* listed above.
2. Aid *bowel eliminations* through the use of colonics or enemas. Other measures to keep bowel movements regular may be needed, but this aid to

eliminations is important to the kidney and bladder
function.

3. The *diet* should be given special attention. In
reading 3050—1 Cayce said:

> . . . there should not be a great deal of meat.
> Never any hog meat, except occasionally a little
> crisp bacon may be taken. Fish, fowl, and lamb
> should be the meats, and these not every day—
> and never fried.

> Leafy vegetables are preferable to the tuberous or
> bulbous nature. A raw salad should be one meal
> each day, or at least part of same. Include raw
> carrots, lettuce, celery, water cress, and especially
> beet tops. These may all be taken raw, if properly
> prepared. For this particular body, these would be
> better in bulk than just taking the juices of same;
> though for some bodies the juices would be better.

> As for breads—only corn bread, using the yellow
> meal, with egg, and whole wheat bread. These are
> preferable.

4. *Osteopathic manipulations* may be needed, depending on the conditions found. In general, they
should be directed to the area of the ninth dorsal
vertebra, which leads to the solar plexus, and to the
lumbar and sacral segments of the spine that inner-
vate the pelvis area.

5. *Hydrotherapy and massage* were suggested in
the readings to improve the circulation—probably
the hepatic circulation mentioned earlier. Glycothymoline packs over the pubic area, heated with a salt
pack that has been heated and then placed over the
Glycothymoline pack, help relieve certain tensions.

6. *Watermelon seed tea or a little Coca-Cola* was
frequently mentioned in the readings as a purifier of
the urine when the urine tends to be acid. To 3390—1,
Cayce said, "In the regular diet, include occasionally
such drinks as Coca-Cola, but with plain water, not
carbonated. These are needed to purify activities in
kidneys and bladder." In reading 540—11, however,
he suggested a little bit of carbonated Coca-Cola,

which would act as the watermelon seed tea, in "purifying or clearing the ducts through the kidneys, and thus reduce the general forces and influences there."

Within these six categories might be listed also the comment that Cayce made to a gentleman who had a urinary-tract stone. In discussing his diet, he noted that chewing the food well supplies the salivary-gland activity that produces the "lactics" or alkalinity as food enters the system. It is always a good rule to remember, especially in those conditions where there is an overacidity.

We have also used—as a counterirritant in the bladder area—another special procedure. After the bladder is massaged thoroughly with a mixture compounded of equal parts of mutton tallow, sprits of turpentine, spirits of camphor, and compound tincture of benzoin, a heated salt pack is applied to the same area, making it hot enough to be comfortable but not so hot as to burn the body.

Prostate

The prostate is part of this general area and can be looked at as part of the bladder and urethra anatomy, for it nearly surrounds the urethra as the latter makes its way out of the bladder. We have always treated enlarged prostates by finger massage at intervals of several days to a week. The six suggestions discussed above are also helpful to the prostate, but exercises are especially helpful.

Dr. Harold Reilly is a legend in the story of Edgar Cayce's life and readings. Many times he was sent patients from the solitude of Cayce's altered state of consciousness. Reilly, now in his eighties, is still giving people high-class physical therapy as he journeys between Virginia Beach and his home in New Jersey. He also directs the fortunes of the Physical Therapy Research Division of the Edgar Cayce Foundation. It is always a pleasure to report on one of his simple remedies—which you might find very useful in the case of prostatitis. In a letter to a friend of mine in the Houston area, he suggested striking the buttocks with doubled-up fists rather sharply about twelve times, three times daily. And, as an additional help:

> Lie on a blanket on the floor (not the bed). Bring knees up and lift the buttocks up and down hitting the floor with a little force (not too much at first) in order to create a vibration through the pelvic region, four times daily to start with and then four times twice a day a bit later. Then increase the "bumps" until you are doing it eight bumps twice a day. Take a month to reach the eight by adding one bump per week, see?

That is Reilly, not Cayce.

Another exercise coming out of the Cayce readings themselves is: stand erect. As you gradually raise your hands to a position directly above your head, rise up to the tips of your toes, trying to stay on tiptoe. Hold your breath until you start to return to the beginning position, letting it out gradually, as you become erect with your hands at your sides.

Urinary Retention

There are obviously many ways of bringing healing to the body. These two different solutions to the problem of urinary retention are a good example. And, as I see these things happen, I always remember the Cayce admonition that healing is bringing a consciousness of the Divine to the awareness of the forces within the body. It's a principle of therapy, not just specifics, that becomes the important thing when treating the human body.

A man who had locomotor ataxia was given a reading back in 1930. He was unable to void; and, for some reason, those attending him were unable to catheterize him. Cayce saw this as a tendency to create a stricture in the neck of the bladder, and gave the following information:

> . . . We would apply as this, added to those packs that have aided the kidneys but not relieved same:

Take into the mouth a piece of resin, about the size of a pea. Let this dissolve, or chew same and swallow that as is created with the salivary reactions by the keeping or holding of same in the mouth. Also prepare about a tablespoonful of pure hog lard, with a level teaspoonful of spirits of turpentine, and make into a poultice, or cloth, and keep *heated* across the body, above the neck of the bladder. This will *relieve* the pressure at the present.

2504–9

Thirteen years later, a woman reported that she had read this particular reading. Her father had been injured in a fall and was in serious condition and was unable to void, so she had him hold a small piece of resin in his mouth; he got the same kind of relief that case 2504 obtained, almost immediately.

Some of my most interesting experiences come from the older generation. One particular patient doesn't act as old as most people think an eighty-two-year-old should. He is still actively working, has a twinkle in his eyes most of the time, and is clearly interested in his health. He awoke one Saturday morning unable to empty his bladder. The acute retention did not subside, despite attempts at refraining from water, taking in an excess of water, and finally drinking a couple of beers, which made him experience excruciating pain. Finally, he told me, he decided that he would use some of the pressure-point therapy he had read about somewhere—he just wasn't going to see me or go to the emergency room. To him, this meant the hospital, and surgery, and that he was *not* going to allow! So he started massaging his ankles between the malleoli and the os calcis. He said: "I didn't rub them once. I massaged those ankles for half a day!" Suddenly he had the urge to urinate, and he proceeded to void three and a half quarts of urine. I checked his prostate nearly four days after the event, and his prostate was normal, but he told me that his stream of urine was better than it had been since he was a

young man. What caused his urinary retention I still
do not know. He had no infection, either.

An interesting aspect to this story is that the areas
of the ankle that he massaged are well supplied with
acupuncture points on both the kidney and the bladder meridians, and he undoubtedly worked with kidney point #7, which is the point of tonification for
this meridian and is used when there is retention of
urine. We found this kind of massage very helpful
for several of our patients over the years, but not all
were successful in relieving the urinary retention. A
man in his early sixties with an enlarged prostate
worked hard at it, but he still needed the surgical
assistance of our urology consultant, who performed
the needed transurethral resection.

The massage, in all these cases, was in the area of
the ankle, between the os calcis and the malleoli—
and the response, given a persistent approach to the
problem, was nearly always encouraging. Recently I
received another letter from a close friend of one of
our patients from out of town, who told her own
story of urinary retention. "For a month," she said,
"I had had a bladder infection, which reached a
crisis when I was completely unable to void, and was
taken to the hospital emergency room and later admitted as a patient, completely dependent on cathe-
terization." For nine days, she received medication,
catheterizations, and consultation with a urologist,
a gynecologist, a neurologist, an internist, and a
psychiatrist. All opinions led down the same road,
and she was operated on and given a Bonomo
catheter, indwelling through a suprapubic opening.
She used this for six days, becoming more depressed
steadily, until her friend told her about the massage
business.

Six hours of massage about the ankles (and later
in other locations) brought about her first spontaneous flow of urine. She continued faithfully with her
massages,

> . . . and each succeeding day I was able to void
> with a little less straining. Meantime, my doctor
> told me to drain the residual urine by the catheter

and measure it after each voiding. When the residual amounts were less than two ounces for a twenty-four-hour period, he removed the Bonomo catheter (four days after I started the pressure-point therapy) and I steadily improved day by day. Now, three weeks later, I am voiding normally although still on medication, because my blood sedimentation rate is still elevated, and there is still discomfort in the urethral area on voiding. I call myself 93% well.

Acupuncture was never mentioned in the Cayce readings. Perhaps it was because there was no one around to give the treatments. However, I have always maintained that any therapy, if it is administered with understanding of and hope in the spiritual nature of man, becomes a building and constructive force. But the patient has to become part of that process. In line with that concept, surgery, X-ray therapy, medicines, physical therapy, prayer, or the laying on of hands brings into the body an awareness that spells healing.

Kidney Stones

The information from the Cayce readings on kidney stones has not been adequately researched or used, but there are interesting bits of information that give insights into the process and its resolution.

One individual who was apparently passing a stone—or trying to—was told to add half a pint of spirits of turpentine to one and a half quarts of hot water. Then cloths were to be dipped in the solution, wrung out, and applied to the lower abdomen, and were to be changed often. Cayce continued:

We find that the application of the turpentine stupes over the area as indicated would offer a means for causing a disintegrating of the stone sufficient for its passage without operative forces; because of the very nature of the penetrating influences of the turpentine.

843–5

Much of what has already been discussed for use in the urinary-tract problems also applies to kidney stones, and it is the position of these readings that most stones can be dissolved without surgery, although evidence that this is the case has not yet been forthcoming at the clinical level.

Nephritis

Using acupuncture—along with a variety of other added therapies—I have watched two different individuals, both males in their twenties, with nephritis, or an inflammation of the kidneys, improve from the point where kidney dialysis was inevitable, in the minds of their attending specialists. Their laboratory tests for blood urea nitrogen and creatinine moved back toward normal. One of the patients, still under therapy, now has completely normal tests on kidney function. The other is aimed in the right direction. It is always difficult to tell what it is that brings a person back to a better state of health when many modalities of therapy are used. But it may be like assessing which one of the fourteen or fifteen basketball players on a championship team was instrumental in making them champions. Is it really one person, or must all of them work together? Perhaps the same question can be asked when it comes to the healing of the human body, for there are many forces of physiology at work, and they either cooperate and coordinate in their activity, or they don't become body champions.

Chapter Twenty One
THE SKIN

The covering of the human body is at the same time necessary, convenient, frequently beautiful, and certainly the largest organ of the body. It is also the site of the greatest number of difficulties—probably because it is on the outside and thereby is most easily affected. The skin is the first line of defense for the body, repelling injury most often. It is affected by our attitudes and emotions when we least suspect them. It is also harmed or aided most seriously by the kind of diet we follow; and it responds to problems of elimination by breaking out in a variety of ways. It grows warts, moles, cancers, and a host of other unidentified objects that frequently receive first aid treatment.

One A.R.E. member wrote to me about a large mole located on his neck right where the collar kept irritating it. He used castor oil on a Band-aid—and, with repeated applications, it started to shrink. "I kept up the swabbing," he reported, "then by the end of the second week, it was very dry with a thin strand holding on. A few days later it fell off and hasn't since come back."

Another intrepid soul had a plantar wart on each foot. He took suggestions from the Cayce readings and used hydrochloric acid on the warts, but they only grew larger. Then, while visiting the A.R.E. library in Virginia Beach, he did some research in the readings and found suggestions about spirits of camphor and sodium bicarbonate. Two weeks of daily treatment to the warts, which had by then grown to an inch in diameter, and they were almost gone. He also had a 3/16-inch conical-shaped skin lesion, which I think must have been an epithelioma, located on his left cheek. Using the same combination he had used on the plantar wart, the growth receded but did not disappear. When he stopped the treatment, the growth reappeared, so he now tried soaking baking soda with castor oil, and using Band-aids to hold the mixture to the skin. In about two weeks, the growths subsided to one tiny, hard spot. Continuing to apply the castor oil-soda mixture as a massage without Band-aids for about two months more, the skin eventually returned to normal.

One of our cooperating M.D.s, Eileen O'Farrell, reported to us that she has found success in treating warts simply with Atomidine; and from the Cayce readings comes this interesting observation:

Q-7: What should I do about the mole on my neck, on which the doctor put some acid for removal?

A-7: Not anything in the present. As those properties suggested begin to take effect, and there are adjustments in the circulation, we find that these will gradually take away the conditions.

We would keep same soft with a little of an equal combination of Mutton Tallow (melted), Spirits of Turpentine and Spirits of Camphor; not so much put on the area of the mole itself as the area about it, so that it will be absorbed by the effect of the properties through the radiation, see?

2426-1

Dermatology in the Cayce readings becomes a much different thing from what I was taught in medical school. I now see the skin as an organ of elimination and protection, a unit that must be coordinated with the other organs of elimination—the lungs, the kidneys, the liver, and the intestines—in order that it stay healthy and able to do its job. The skin has consciousness, like other parts of the body, and wants to perform its role in a creative, helpful manner. However, the skin is affected by food and by aberrant neurological impulses that frequently require manipulative therapy for correction; and it is a major part of the structure of the body, presenting to the outside world a symbolic story of what is happening in the inner world and consciousness of the person who wears the skin. Since the skin is a reflection of events that are happening in other parts of the body, as well as the outside environment, we would suspect that it would respond to therapeutic treatments aimed at other systems, other functions, as well as to those remedies applied locally.

Acne

Acne, the scourge of both the male and the female teenager, is found in the Cayce materials to be caused by a thinning of the walls of the intestines, which allows the bloodstream to become polluted as it serves both the intestinal walls and the skin. While it is not stated clearly whether emotions or heredity initiate this problem, it does become rather clear that blockages in the autonomic nervous system are partially the cause and frequently require osteopathic manipulative treatments. It is also true that diet becomes a major factor in causing acne; and diet is the constant recommendation in the readings, as well as for those individuals whom I have personally treated for acne.

Often, in an effort to aid the regeneration of the thinned walls of the intestine, I prescribe a teaspoon of a prepared mixture of perhaps one tablespoon each of Rochelle salts, sulfur, and cream of tartar, mixed very well—preferably with a mortar and pestle. This is to be taken once a day before meals with a glass of water. After a period of two or three weeks, I have the patient get some osteopathic treatments.

One simple and highly effective treatment for acne is simply massaging castor oil into the affected parts of the skin before retiring each night. I always suggest a change of diet, also, but even when it is not seriously followed, the castor oil aids greatly. Perhaps the lymphatic drainage—enhanced by the use of the castor oil—provides the therapy in such an instance.

The diet I would suggest would be one that is free of most of the elements that might cause skin trouble. Realizing that there are always exceptions to every rule, I recommend the following:

1. Take a yeast cake or a packet of dry yeast and blend into eight ounces of tomato or V-8 juice. You may use other juices if you wish. A dash of lime juice and worcester sauce adds a little tang in the V-8 mix. Take once a day for ten days. Then stop for a week and repeat.
2. Obtain some Coca-Cola syrup from a soda fountain. Take one teaspoon in a glass of *plain* water once or twice a day.
3. No chocolate, sugars, ice cream, pastries, pie, or candy.

4. No carbonated drinks, including diet drinks. No beer or ale.
5. No pork or ham. *Crisp* bacon allowed, however.
6. Limit starches to *one* per meal: bread, rice, potato, spaghetti, corn, etc. No white bread.
7. No fried foods. This includes Fritos and potato chips.
8. Vegetables are good for you. Have plenty of salads, vegetable soup, cooked vegetables. Salad dressing is okay.
9. Fruits are fine in season, except raw apple, strawberry, and banana.
10. Meats: especially recommended are lamb, fish, fowl. *Lean* beef is all right.
11. Milk (skim), eggs, and cheese are allowed.

Warts

Warts in the human body sometimes create a major problem for those who seem to be particularly susceptible. It has been known for decades now that there are viruses present in warts, and many people regard viruses as the cause of this condition. Yet, no one has clearly explained the origin or destiny of viruses and whether they simply cause trouble or are there as the result of trouble.

In the Edgar Cayce readings, a completely different picture of warts is described—a story that seems to say that warts come about because of living processes that have gone awry and that need correction:

It is the accumulation of cellular forces attempting to act themselves. Or, as we see, every atom of the body is as a whole universe or an element in itself. It either coordinates or it makes for disruptive forces by its activity being expelled from the system through the activity of the eliminating system; and as it accumulates it gathers those things about it and is not absorbed. Hence we have them as moles or warts.

759-9

It might be observed that human consciousness

has a great deal to do with the formation of warts, as well as with their elimination from the body. At the same time, the whole immune system is related, in function and in response, to the consciousness of the body's owner. How else could we explain the curing of warts by hypnosis, or by the touch of a special person, or by simple suggestion, or by what we call spontaneous remission? These things certainly have happened and have been reported in medical journals.

My own brother, John, had a problem with warts. His son had been urging him to try castor oil, but everyone in my family seemingly must follow his or her individual urge to be creative. So, John reflected a bit, remembered how we had talked about iodine as being a curative agent, and decided to use tincture of iodine on his warts. He treated them just a few times, simply applying the iodine to the tops of the warts, and before long the warts had disappeared. There are indeed many ways to remove these annoying growths.

I recently found a pigmented mole neatly folded in a piece of plastic and stapled to the front of a letter from one of our patients. My correspondent noted one night that the large mole that had been present on her husband's back for as long as she could remember seemed to be enlarging in size. Their internist told them that they need not have it removed immediately, but that they should keep a close watch on it. One night soon after, she

suddenly had the urge to put castor oil on the mole and cover it with a Band-aid soaked in the oil. Don agreed that it would be an interesting experiment although neither of us remember Cayce saying anything about moles and castor oil. I did this until April 13, when Don was out of town several days on business. Last night I noticed the Band-aid still intact and suggested we return to our nightly care of it. When I removed the Band-aid, I noticed the mole was loose around the edges. I lifted one corner and the shrunken remains came off easily—beneath it was fresh pink skin!

The whole process took only twenty days. The pathology specimen arrived in my hands just a couple of days after that. Our laboratory report indicated that this mole had melanin in it, typical of a mole, and there was no evidence of malignancy.

Scars

Scars are dealt with rather thoroughly in the Cayce readings. Cayce suggested a variety of treatment combinations: olive oil and tincture of myrrh alternated with camphorated oil; camphorated oil by itself; camphorated oil, witch hazel, and mineral oil (as part of acne treatment); camphorated oil, lanolin, and peanut oil; cocoa butter and olive oil; Epson salt packs followed by cocoa butter rubbed in; and olive oil and camphorated oil equal parts, to mention just a few. It should be noted that in the days when the readings were given, camphorated oil was made with olive oil and a bit of the crude camphor, while today it is made mostly with cottonseed oil.

Cayce stated in 487–17 that "any scar tissue detracts from the general physical health of a body," and he consistently recommended measures such as those to remove the scar. The physiological removal is through the eliminatory systems, bit by bit, but it must be done in decency and order. He suggested this very factually:

. . . Do not break up the deposits of the scar tissue, or calcium deposits, more than can be regularly or naturally done by increasing the eliminations; that is, do not break up more of the scar tissue than can be eliminated from the body. These should be eliminated not only through the respiratory and perspiratory system but through the alimentary canal. After each period of using the Packs, epsom salts, massage the cocoa butter about the foot and gradually make those changes that will cause a better position of the structural portions of toe, the instep and the Achilles bursa.

4003–1

We have found results to be highly satisfactory if the patient is willing to use the scar lotion persistently and consistently over a long enough period of time. But we never had results like that obtained by one of our correspondents who was injured in a ski accident in January 1972. The knee suffered torn and crushed cartileges, which were removed by surgery one month later. Pain continued severely for six weeks, then gradually lessened. One year of therapy allowed her to flex the knee ninety degrees, and she noticed that there was much "hard" tissue around the knee joint proper.

In October 1973, she started using a scar preparation made up of camphorated olive oil 80%, peanut oil 18%, and lanolin 2%. At first, she applied it only to the surgical scars, but then, before retiring one night, she decided to use it over the entire knee. When she did so, she reported that she felt the knee become loose around the areas of induration or hardening. The next day, she repeated the procedure while noting that the kneecap was movable and the tissues were soft. After the third day's treatment, she noticed that the knee was normal in size, and she was able to flex the knee normally as compared to the other leg. Pain and tightness were gone as she used her knee now. The improvement lasted and normalcy resulted.

The most common formula for compounding the scar lotion is simply two ounces of camphorated oil, one-half teaspoon of dissolved or melted lanolin, and one ounce of peanut oil. It is suggested that the oil be used daily until the scar has become so faint that it cannot be noticed. One story I received from a Cedar Rapids girl tells about the use of this lotion on a surgical scar:

> We started my fifteen-year-old sister using the scar lotion last summer on a 5½-by-1¼-inch surgical scar on her back. Within the first three days of application, a hole left by a catheter (in the scar) rapidly filled in with new tissue or skin, although it had been very slow in healing

before. The scar is now somewhat smaller, but, more importantly, is losing its whiteness and turning more towards normal skin in color and texture.

Blood Poisoning

Lymphangitis and cellulitis were called blood poisoning when I was a child. I remember how deathly afraid my parents were of such a condition getting a start. Russ Simondson, an old friend of mine, found excellent responses to one Cayce suggestion for lymphangitis Where red streaks mark the lymphatic channels that have become seriously infected from a wound—usually on the hand, foot, arm, or leg—Russ uses a pack made out of salt moistened with spirits of turpentine covered and bound around the extremity. The pack should not cover the wound itself, and it need not cover the farthest extension of the lymphangitis. Rather, it should be just two or three inches distance from the wound itself between the wound and the heart. Russ found that such a pack cleared up not only the red streak that we call lymphangitis but also the original cellulitis or inflammation where the wound originated.

Bee stings were found to be treated in the same manner as lymphangitis. The bee sting area itself should not be covered, but the pack should be placed, again, near to the bee sting, just a few inches away.

Pruritis

The excellent result experienced in this next story may have been due to multilevel therapy, or it may have been simply the effect brought into being by the continued application of patience. Or it may simply have been elm water. We probably will never really know the cause—but the response is no doubt a major factor in making life a really enjoyable experience for a seventeen-year-old girl. She was fifteen when she was taken to a cooperating doctor in the Edgar Cayce Foundation Chiropractic Research Division. Her problem was a serious generalized pruritis (itching) associated with a chronic dermatitis, and she had been under the care of various specialists her entire life. Her therapy program was a strict diet avoiding meats, milk, dairy products, cereals, starches, and sweets. She was given saffron tea regularly, and she was treated with regular manipulations. After three months she showed no improvement. The parents, at the suggestion of their doctor, called the Clinic, and we suggested only the addition of elm water (slippery elm bark in water). Another five months passed with several flare-ups, but then a gradual improvement was noted. Now, after another year of continuing the same regimen, the mother writes that "our daughter is now able to lead an almost normal life and is so much improved."

In the readings, a forty-eight-year-old man (437–7) had been suffering constant, severe itching for many weeks. The causes were enumerated as a thinning of the walls of the jejunum, a section of the small intestine, due to lack of proper "reactions." The resulting condition was a fouling-up, so to speak, of the blood supply as it coursed through the walls of the small intestine. This, in turn, brought about a disturbed circulation and a subcutaneous irritation interpreted as itching. In short, it was a problem of eliminations. A diet was suggested, along with small quantities of olive oil by mouth and some local applications, and osteopathic adjustments.

In still another reading, the first two paragraphs are of special interest as to the cause of itching. The subject, a twenty-four-year-old man, complained of intractable itching most of the time and had been a puzzle to his doctors:

> As we find, there are those disturbances in the chemical processes of the body through the lack of proper eliminations or drainages being set up through the whole system, so that poisons which should be carried off through the alimentary canal, or through the activity of the kidneys and bladder are at times eliminated through the respiratory system.

These, by those activities through the body cause
chemical changes; and these have been made for
pressures in the segments along the spine where
minor lesions have formed, especially in the areas
from the first of the dorsals, or first the third
cervical, then through the upper dorsal and the
area of the ninth dorsal. . . .

5157–1

Emotions, Sex and Skin

Emotions, sex, and skin are related. One patient
of mine had a chronic, stubborn case of dry inflammation of the skin, or eczema, which paralleled an
unsatisfactory, sometimes stormy love affair. She
had literally exhausted the drug store supply of
medicines, several clinics, many dermatologists, and
the nutrition literature, all to no avail. In her words:

So, during these four years I've had a rather see-
saw-y relationship with a guy. And when we broke
up and I was away from him, my eczema seemed
to clear up. . . . But I have learned one thing. It
wasn't due to him personally but my mixed emotions about sex. When I get uptight about sex, my
hands literally "bloom" one to two days later.

Cayce had much to say about these relationships.
In one reading, he suggested that the subject, a
forty-four-year-old engineer, read and study Exodus
and chapter 30 of Deuteronomy (applied in the terms
of Psalm 23), and he also recommended some interesting physical therapy treatments. Mr. Cayce's final
admonition at the end of the reading was:

As we find, there are disturbances with this body.
Much of these, however, are tied up with the emotional natures of the body. And here we find some
of those conditions of which many bodies should
be warned—the opening of centers in the body-
spiritual without correctly directing same, which
may oft lead to wrecking of the body-physical and

sometimes mental. Know where you are going before you start out, in analyzing spiritual and mental and material things.

This is not belittling the seeking of knowledge, neither is it advising individuals—or this individual—to seek knowledge. But knowledge without the use of same still remains, as in the beginning, sin. And be sure your sins will find you out!

Here we have an emotional body well versed in the study of meditation, the study of transmission of thought, with the ability to control others.

Don't control others, suppose thy God controlled thee without thy will? What would you become, or what would you have been?

But you were made in the image of thy Creator, to be a companion with Him—not over someone else, but a companion with thy brother and not over thy brother. Hence do not act that way, because ye have the greater ability or greater knowledge of control of others.

Q-1: Is the focal center of the disease in the brain or some other part of the body?

A-1: As indicated, it is in those centers—the seven centers of the body—where sympathetic and cerebrospinal coordinate the more; 1st, 2nd and 3rd cervical; 1st and 2nd dorsal; 5th and 6th dorsal; 9th dorsal; 11th and 12th dorsal; and through the lumbar and sacral areas. These are the sources. This is not an infection—it is the lack of coordination between the impulses of the mental self and the central nerve and blood supply.

Q-2: Are there any organic changes due to the disease?

A-2: All of the organic changes are due to this condition, of lack of coordination.

Q-3: Does sexual expression or repression cause this condition, or have any effect on same?

A-3: This was a part of the beginnings of it; for when lyden [Leydig] glands are opened, which are in the gonads—or the centers through which the expression of generation begins, they act directly upon the centers through the body. Unless these find expression they disintegrate, or through thy assocation cause dis-association in impulse and the central or body-nerves.

Q-4: Are there any mental attitudes involved in the cause of this disease?

A-4: As indicated.

Do as outlined—we will have the results, according to thy faith and thy works; not by faith alone but by faith AND works.

3428-1

Puncture Wounds

Some time ago I treated a cat bite with castor oil packs kept on continuously—without heat—for sixteen to twenty hours daily. This was in addition to the usual therapies. The hand and wrist cleared up remarkably and quickly—much more so than had been my experience in the past. Since then, when we have had minor puncture wounds from working with our palm trees or other desert-type vegetation, we have had excellent results using castor oil rubbed into the skin several times a day. In fact, we have not had one infection using castor oil. Once or twice we have had to go in after a couple of days and take out a piece of the vegetation that had imbedded itself in the tissues, but no infection was there, and rapid healing came about.

Our youngest son brought home from school a rat whose career as a laboratory animal had ended. Well, David took good care of the rat, but at our annual New Year's party and meditation for the kids and their parents, someone tipped over Zorba's cage. She was not wild, but she was scared at all the humans reaching for her to place her back in her home. My wife, Gladys, exercising the best techniques from her past incarnation as a vet, picked up Zorba and placed her back in her cage. Zorba, however, was still suffering from an adrenal response of fear, and just before Gladys let go, Zorba reached around and bit Gladys on the finger. While the story is interesting, the important part of the event was that castor oil, rubbed into the rat bite over the next two days, caused the wound to heal without complications or pain. It further illustrates how we have used this oil, derived from the bean of the *Ricinus communis*, on puncture wounds, bites, and minor cuts and bruises, with a very high degree of success.

Psoriasis

Psoriasis is a chronic but noncontagious skin disease characterized by inflammation and white, scaly patches. Recent advances in the art and science of medicine bring psoriasis and peritoneal dialysis together for the first time. Researchers at the University of Missouri at Columbia report unusually promising responses in therapy of the psoriasis patient.

Dr. Zbylut J. Twardowski noted a beneficial response in psoriasis patients undergoing peritoneal dialysis at the Hospital for Miners in Bytom, Poland (*Medical World News*, April 17, 1978). During a sabbatical at Columbia, he urged Drs. Nolph and Anderson, heads of the renal and dermatological departments, to do a pilot study. A preliminary report on sixteen patients was very encouraging. "The first patient we treated had been unable to move her joints or sit down, had been unemployed, and was threatening suicide," Dr. Nolph said. "Her lesions cleared up with just four treatments, and she has been free of the disease for ten months."

Their working hypothesis is that in psoriasis there is some organic compound or metabolite—yet to be identified—that is not excreted by the kidney, yet is small enough to be dialyzed or separated out. Perhaps the kidney filters it, but the substance is then reabsorbed just as the kidney reabsorbs glucose, according to Dr. Nolph. Over years the "metabolite" builds up in body fluids and finally reaches the level necessary for psoriasis to start. Then, when the patient is dialyzed, the fluid levels of this "metabolite" drop below the amount that causes the problem. Although the results thus far are encouraging, the researchers remain cautious, and look for a double-blind study, controlled sufficiently to bind down the conclusions.

It is interesting that these researchers do not deal with the basic cause of the production of the "metabolite," which certainly must underlie the process itself. The substance is just there. There is perhaps nothing wrong with this observation, but it remains as fact that there is an abnormality of function or structure that produces such a metabolite, which, in turn, if it does exist, *does* cause psoriasis, and it does involve the excretory function of the body—since the skin, like the kidneys and the liver and intestine, is an excretory organ.

In the material gathered over the years from the Edgar Cayce psychic readings, psoriasis was a frequent subject of discussion. Dr. Fred Lansford wrote a medical commentary on psoriasis, and the information he supplies is particularly interesting when put into perspective with the work done at Columbia with dialysis. Let me simply quote from three readings that are found in his manuscript:

There are disturbing conditions which prevent the better physical functioning in this body These have to do primarily with an intestinal disorder and the lack of proper coordination in the eliminating systems. There are those conditions, then, in the duodenum and through the jejunum where there are the effects as if there were tiny thinned walls, as if the walls of the duodenum had been smoothed—rather than the folds that should exist with the gastric flow which should come through these areas at periods of digestion. The results are a disturbance in the blood supply and an irritation in the superficial circulation, so that those areas in the epidermis show eliminations that should be carried through the alimentary canal, for these are being eliminated through perspiratory system.

3373–1 (F., 74 yrs.)

Q-1: Is Psoriasis always from the same cause?

A-1: No, but it is more often from the lack of proper coordination in the eliminating systems. At times these pressures may be in those areas disturbing the equilibrium between the heart and liver, or between heart and lungs. But it is always caused by a condition of lack of lymph circulation through alimentary canal and by absorption of such activities through the body.

5016–1 (F., 25 yrs.)

In some times back we had a condition that existed from toxic forces, or by the accumulations through and to the stubborn condition in an *improper* elimination through the alimentary canal. This strain at the time from fecal forces in the system tended to make for a thinning of the walls of the intestines themselves, making a secretion that—having to be taken up by the lymph and emunctories, and the blood being impoverished—produces a rash on the exterior forces of the body at times.

622–1 (M., 29 yrs.)

The Cayce material always seems to see problems in the human body stemming from abnormal physiology that in turn has its origin in attitudes of mind, emotional manners of reacting, or spiritual causes. These always seem to be patterns of reaction that are often so ingrained as to be habitual in nature and poorly understood; and, when manifested in the human body, they become real, they become physical, and they are then called diseases.

The work by the researchers should give those who have psoriasis more hope and certainly more understanding that the various suggestions for therapy as seen in the Cayce material can have a beneificial effect on the skin. All of which leads me to our experiences with patients who have psoriasis. We have seen such individuals cleared up using these Cayce suggestions. There are specific recommendations for therapy of a systemic nature, aiming for (1) an improvement of the functions of assimilation of foods and eliminatory processes; (2) a clearing up of accumulated toxic substances in the circulatory and alimentary systems; and (3) the healing of the intestinal lesions that allow the toxic substances to leak into the circulatory system.

So, using osteopathic manipulations; elm water, yellow saffron, and mullein tea; a basic diet eliminating fats, sweets, and pastries, and adding a great deal of fruits and vegetables; colonics; and an occasional course of triple salts (sulfur, Rochelle salts, and cream of tartar mixed well in equal parts) using one teaspoonful once or twice daily for several days, we have seen great improvements in our psoriasis patients.

Psoriasis is a miserable problem to a twelve-year-old girl. Sally found this out. Her parents took her to dermatologists at the county general hospital where they lived, after she had not improved in three months of U-V ray treatments, bath oils, and a shampoo for her scalp. Under a new regimen of sun lamp, ointments, and Baker's P & S oil, she improved slightly for a while, and then, during this four-month period, the lesions multiplied and worsened. Sally's parents then put her on the diet Cayce prescribed: peanut oil was used locally on the worst of the lesions and on the scalp, and the chamomile, saffron, mullein, and elm teas were used. She rapidly (in two weeks) began to improve, and after a year's therapy is clear of the problem, with the exception of two very small spots on her scalp that seem to be clearing up.

Relief from psoriasis is undoubtedly best pursued through adjustment of the diet. This theme appears over and over again in the Cayce readings and in our own experience. However, other factors can help greatly. Osteopathic treatments were frequently recommended. It takes patience and application of principles while the patience is being utilized. Patience, persistence, and consistency—three words that are found throughout the Cayce readings and tell the story of success.

Scleroderma

Scleroderma is one of a group of what are called collagen diseases or diseases of the connective tissues of the body. Other manifestations of this abnormality in the body are periarteritis nodosa, systemic lupus erythematosus, dermatomyositis, and what may be called variants of polyarteritis. They are often difficult to diagnose and even more difficult to treat. There are a number of readings and lots of suggestions given by Edgar Cayce relative to this very destructive illness.

In 1968, Alan R. Cantwell, Jr., a dermatologist in California, introduced us to the factual information that acid-fast bacteria are present in the skin of scleroderma patients, with his first paper dealing with this information at our first medical symposium in Phoenix. At the same time, he pinned down the accurate medical clairvoyance that Cayce demonstrated so often—for Cayce said in the 1920s that such bacteria were present in the skin of these patients.

Edgar Cayce, however, did not see scleroderma being caused by a bacteria. The disease is a process, and a complicated one, affecting not only the skin but the blood-forming structural areas such as the bone and the lung tissue itself. It is a process that produces a hardening or a clotting of the blood, mainly as a result of the blood itself attempting to bring about coagulation—that creative process within the body that is the building up of new tissue as old tissue normally dies. This is seen most graphically in the skin where the superficial circulation to the various layers of the skin itself is involved in this process. Then, nerves ending in these areas become deadened because of their involvement in the process, which in turn results in acute pain and also reflexes to the autonomic nervous system, which then becomes involved itself. In this manner the organs throughout the body become disturbed.

There are glands within the body—in the case of scleroderma, these being principally the thyroid, the adrenals, and the liver—that become deficient in supplying elements that normally would keep all portions of the skin normal. These glandular elements are necessary in the formation of structure out of energy as Cayce described the event many times in his readings. With these hormones absent, the effect on the glands is, apparently, to produce a tubercle bacillus or germ in the lymphatics of the skin as a direct result of the skin being destroyed and becoming hardened more rapidly than it can be rebuilt. This becomes a "consumptive" condition with an inflammation of the lymph in that area between the outer, the inner, and the most-inner portions of the skin covering.

Far-advanced cases, of course, have nearly all portions of the body involved. Thus, little of the oxygen needed by the body can be met by a malfunctioning respiratory system, and the entire body is put under a greater strain. As these conditions progress, assimilation becomes more difficult and less capable, and the lack of reconstructive activities in the body progressively becomes more acute. The glands, then, are seen as the primary cause leading to a difficult end unless measures are taken to reverse the trend and rebuild the body.

A comprehensive regimen of therapy, as taken from the Cayce readings, would be to use Atomidine and the wet cell battery to work on the glandular system, the nerves, and the bringing into the body those energies needed; a dietary regimen and care for the organs of assimilation to provide that which is needed through the alimentary canal; local therapy of the skin through massages and applications such as castor oil; inhalants to purify the lungs and keep the oxygen supply upgraded; and those other therapies such as colonics and other measures that might be needed for more advanced cases.

The diet to be used is always that of an alkaline-forming or alkaline-ash nature—many leafy vegetables as the main ingredient. Fish, fowl, and lamb are the best proteins, but never fried foods. Vegetable soups and other foods easily assimilated are recommended. Also suggested are vegetables cooked with patapar paper or the equivalent parchment paper that may

be purchased at most health food stores. Meat should
not be cooked with vegetable soups.

Scleroderma, as a disease process, reverses itself
often in a most gratifying manner under the rehabilitative regimen that Cayce suggested. The late Dr.
Frank Dobbins, who retired in Key West from his
years of practice in the New York area, started a
patient on this course of treatment before he left. I
received a letter from the gentleman when he had
found himself without a doctor for several months.
The response was so notable that I thought you
would like to read a few quotes from his letter.

> Before I started these treatments, as a mem-
> ber of the A.R.E. I received the Cayce file on sclero-
> derma and was rubbing my afflicted area with
> castor oil, peanut oil, and olive oil for over a year
> prior to "seeing Dobbins." Before the castor oil
> rubs and packs, my ankles and calves were blood
> red, now they look normal. . . .
>
> I am happy, doctor, to report I seem to have
> reversed the debilitating effect of the scleroderma
> and that areas of my body seem to be free of the
> harshness or much improved. The skin on my
> forearms can be punched and pulled where before
> it felt like stone and had no give. My legs feel
> better, and I am able to walk quite a few blocks
> now before they tire. I also have much less pain in
> my joints and have feeling in my fingertips and
> the soles of my feet. The best thing I can say is
> that my friends and relatives stopped treating me
> as if I was going to die.

Castor oil and scleroderma come together frequently as we treat those individuals who are afflicted with this serious condition. Castor oil packs
are helpful in a variety of ways, one of them being
the softening of the skin locally where they are
applied. In the many readings Cayce gave for people
with this condition. I found the suggestion often
that the skin should be washed with bicarbonate of
soda water prior to the application of the packs of
castor-oil-saturated flannel. Since the soda does an

excellent job of cleansing the skin *after* the packs
are removed, being one of the few things that will
cut the oil itself, I assume that Cayce's suggestion
may have some relationship to the removal of toxins
from the skin before the packs, so these would not
be carried into the body by the use of the heat and
the packs.

Skin Cancers

Skin cancers are bothersome in the early stages,
and, of course, they are life-threatening if not treated
before they spread to other parts of the body. My
purpose here is just to touch on some simple ways
to stop early growth of skin cancers. Sometimes
these are effective, sometimes not—many factors come
into play in the human body in any of the cancers.
Cancer of the skin is certainly a condition that involves all the concepts dealt with in this chapter and
in this book. It cannot be emphasized too strongly
that cancers must be cured locally or removed to call
the therapy adequate. Otherwise, one's very life is
threatened when a cancer metastasizes or spreads
to other parts of the body.

Cancer of the skin seems to develop on the face
and the exposed parts of the arms and hands more
commonly than elsewhere. I have recommended application of castor oil to some of these lesions on a
regular basis daily, while I observe the progress of
the lesion or its disappearance. I had never used
Atomidine topically for these skin problems, although
I have found it useful in treating small irritations of
the skin and minor infections. Recently we received
a letter from one of our correspondents in Birmingham, Alabama, who tells how he treats skin cancers
on his face with Atomidine. He has been bothered
with these for some twenty-five years, having had a
number removed surgically, with X-ray follow-up.
Pathological exam confirmed the malignancy of the
lesions each time.

In the past several years he has taken off in a new
direction. Having read something from the readings

about using Atomidine to stimulate glandular activity, he reasoned that this should take care of the cancer. So, he started using it locally. Let me quote him:

> First the area was cleansed with "Sayman's soap for oily skin" to remove the oil and allow the Atomidine to come in contact with the skin. Then a drop of Atomidine was applied with an eyedropper and the drop allowed to remain on the cancer until it dried. This was done morning and night. The only discomfort was a mild stinging until the Atomidine dried. Some swelling and redness occurred over an area about the size of a quarter, but this subsided in a few days. Treatment was continued for a week or so. Careful examination would disclose in some instances a small slight depression remaining, but essentially there was no scar left. I have removed ten or twelve by this method with no ill effects.

As an alternative to surgery, my correspondent finds this to be acceptable. When Atomidine stays on the skin for thirty seconds to a minute, it starts to burn a bit—not severely. But no harm came about, and I've never found it to be harmful when I have used it on the skin.

Castor oil has been used widely in instances of skin cancer. One doctor who has worked closely with the Cayce remedies reports:

> With regard to the skin . . . a man about 68 years old had a mean-looking lesion on his ear which was probably an early squamous cell carcinoma; biopsy was not done. This lesion had been present for years. The patient has had basal cell carcinoma removed from the area of the left ear somewhat near this particular lesion. At any rate, after two weeks of the castor oil and camphorated oil, the lesion disappeared and has not recurred. The treatment was started in December of 1969.

> Another patient, a woman of 61, had a lesion inside her ear in the external auditory meatus,

which was rough and scaly, and she used the
castor oil-camphorated oil. The lesion disappeared
and has maintained its absence after about three
weeks of treatment. No recurrence since April 22.
This lesion had been bleeding a bit, and this I
think makes the result with the oil combination
even more dramatic.

Other Skin Conditions

Dermatitis of the hand had been the constant
complaint of a friend of mine. The palm of her hand
had not been clear of a very bothersome rash for
twelve years. She had been to many doctors and had
used literally dozens of medicines, but no real response had been noted. She read about the way
witch hazel is suggested to be used in the Cayce
readings, and she started applying it to her hand
several times a day. Within just two weeks, the hand
was greatly improved and was nearing normalcy.
Witch hazel has its origin from a small shrub called
Hamamelis virginiana. The leaves and bark are used
to make this old-time remedy. There is an alcoholic
and a nonalcoholic form of the medication. It has been
used internally in dysentery, but it is most often
used as an astringent or as a wash for burns,
bruises, skin irritations, and other forms of external
inflammation.

Canker sores, fever blisters, aphthous ulcers—all
seem to be closely related even though given different names. In 1972, Dr. Harvey Rose reported on a
series of cases where he used Atomidine first, applied to the lesion, leaving it on for thirty seconds,
then applying Glycothymoline to the treatment area.
This produces almost instant relief from the discomfort, and he reported healing occurring even in
resistant cases in one to three days.

Footnote to Healing

To be patient, persistent, and consistent while
applying a therapy to the human body—whether it
be for cancer of the skin or for a sinus condition—

calls forth from the person the need to agree with the suggestion given him, to consent that it is okay, to allow things to happen, and to accept the results as they come into being.

Chapter Twenty Two
THE HEART AND VASCULAR SYSTEM

When something goes wrong with the heart or part of the vascular system as a whole, it is often a crisis event. However, such an occurrence is the result of a sequence of events that have developed over an extended period of time. For instance, it takes a period of several years to build up enough cholesterol plaques in the coronary arteries of the heart to set the stage for a typical coronary clotting or thrombosis; and then there are the years that follow, sometimes lasting an entire lifetime, where care must be exercised to prevent recurrence of such a heart attack.

The concern of this book, and this chapter in particular, is to provide concepts and methods that, when applied, act to prevent such serious illnesses, or aid in the regeneration of the body after an event like a coronary takes places. In addition, this book also attempts to present aids that can be applied in one's home and that tend to reverse other, much more common problems afflicting most of us at one time or another.

It must be understood that all disease we ecounter as human beings represents a time-oriented process of deranged physiology of some kind. In other words, the source of the problem lies within our own very being, whether it stems from emotional turmoil that lowers bodily resistance, leading to infection, or from an injury that has a karmic flavor to it and that sets up certain adverse neurological activities ending up in a disease process like multiple sclerosis. Then, in order to prevent a disease from happening or in order to rehabilitate and regenerate the body after a disease occurs, one must, under both circumstances, employ the principles of therapy that enable the body to reverse its direction, correcting the injury or restoring the integrity of the bodily system that builds immunity and prevents infection.

Angina Pectoris

From the information in the Cayce readings, angina pectoris or severe pain in the chest results from a series of physiological malfunctions involving the assimilation of food, the eliminations from the body of "used and refused forces," the balance of the circulatory system, and the relationship between the cerebrospinal and the autonomic nervous systems. It also involves the coordination and close interrelationship between the liver, the lungs, and the heart. Therapy is keyed to function, meaning the application of certain *physical procedures* to bring about desired results, even if one has been unable to do the same thing through activities of the mind and the spirit.

(1) In all cases, "the poisons *must* be taken away." A high colonic once a month perhaps could be taken as the standard, with attention being given to bring about normal daily eliminations; proper urinary function; exercise to make the body sweat regularly (exercise to be started slowly and gradually increased); and improvement of body breathing habits. These procedures all aid in bringing about a balanced elimination for the whole body.

(2) The diet should be a normal basic diet. Wholegrain breads should be used but no white sugar or white flour products. No fried or processed foods. Lots of fresh vegetables and fresh fruit. Cooked vegetables are acceptable. No pork, and beef only occasionally. Fish, fowl, and lamb are acceptable. Cayce suggests that no concentrated vitamins should be added; however, if one feels he is deficient in vitamins from the foods that must be used and that are available, vitamins can be added to aid the body.

(3) Atomidine was suggested in the readings to aid in balancing the circulatory system.

(4) Massage of the entire lower extremities was frequently advised to increase circulation in the feet and legs. One combination of oils suggested was:

Olive oil	1 oz.
Compound tincture of benzoin	1 oz.
Oil of mustard	5 drops

(5) Osteopathic treatments or deep massage, especially to the upper back, were frequently recommended, sometimes to be carried out over a long period of time. For one individual, Cayce suggested weekly treatments for thirty weeks, while to another he recommended treatments twice a week for ten weeks.

Angina does not always come before a heart attack, but the general principles of prevention or care of the anginal patient certainly have a direct relationship to coronary atherosclerosis, or the buildup of hardened areas inside the coronary vessels of the heart. The atherosclerosis found in the arteries can be reduced and made to disappear, much like it was formed in the first place—by reversing the procedures that control the depositing of calcium and cholesterol as plaques or hardened areas in the first place.

For years there was no "hard," scientific evidence that these plaques could be reversed. However, in 1978, a study was published showing that there can actually be a change for the better in atherosclerosis. David Blankenhorn reports that his group performed femoral arteriograms in patients with Type II and Type IV hyperlipoproteinemia, using digital-image processing to obtain a computerized estimate of atherosclerotic-lesion size. They made initial measurements, then placed twenty-five patients on an appropriate diet-drug program, repeating the arteriograms in thirteen months. Lesion size regressed in fourteen patients and did not progress in four others (*Circulation* 57 [1978]: 355–61).

Every physician who has used a nutrition-and-exercise program with patients having obvious disease of the large arteries has observed clinically that the function—which to a great extent mirrors the structure—has improved remarkably. In my work, utilizing concepts from the Cayce readings in the practice of medicine, I have seen this kind of response frequently; but it remains for the research centers to confirm what one's clinical sense cries out loudly must be the case. One of the Cayce readings gives a body-mind-spirit rationale to the concept of regeneration of the body or regression of plaques:

> One should consider, as in this body, that the physical body in its creation was and is given the ability to reproduce itself. Thus each organ, each portion of the body secretes, from the physical, the mental and the spiritual life, that needed to reproduce itself for a growth to better conditions— or the realm for which it prepares itself. When these activities break down, these have to be supplied or they call on other portions of the organism—and thus disintegration begins in one form or another.
>
> 3337–1

Strokes

Other common diseases of the vascular system— strokes, high blood pressure, and thrombophlebitis, to mention a few—are, in a true sense, end products of a disturbed metabolism, a condition that could have been prevented through using the same concepts of care already described in this chapter. Underlying the production of a stroke, for instance, are accumulations of poisons in the system from poor eliminations, improper diet, and malfunctioning assimilation of foods. On top of this are probably superimposed elevated blood pressure or stresses that have not been compensated for; and the result is a major life-threatening crisis.

In considering the physiology involved in a stroke, it is important to remember that the functioning of the extremities and the locomotor facilities (muscular abilities) is not entirely dependent upon the brain and the direction it gives. If the locomotor centers of control, the nerve centers in the spinal cord and the sympathetic ganglia, are brought back to a balance after a stroke, full function should be able to be restored, provided that injury to the brain is not severe enough to bring about death. Balance of function among the circulatory system, the sympathetic nervous system, and the locomotor centers is a critical factor. Four basic fundamentals of therapy need to be followed:

(1) Keep circulation from progressing to a more toxic and unbalanced condition by using tub baths, sweats, colonics, massages, etc.

(2) Use a diet of light foods at first, such as juices, coddled egg and toast, or well-cooked foods. No fried foods, no pork, and no white flour or white sugar substances are permitted. Fish, fowl, or lamb are used for meats. Vegetable juices are always good.

(3) Remove pressures on the sympathetic centers and the locomotor centers with osteopathic treatments, physical therapy, or deep massage.

(4) Promote attitudinal and emotional change that aids the body in rebuilding to normal. This relates not only to the efforts of the stroke patient himself, but to members of his family and the assistance of outside professionals.

It would be well to study the A.R.E.'s Circulating File on Apoplexy, which is simply an older term for *stroke*. The file gives more detail than can be offered here, but the principles are the same. Cayce may seem repetitive in his suggestions, but is consistent in saying that correction will come about only when one applies *therapy that is constructive in a consistent manner, with persistence and patience.*

Thrombophlebitis

Thrombophlebitis, or blood clots in the vein, is sometimes a serious condition. It can let loose a portion of a blood clot, which can then flow through the venous return to the heart and lodge in the lung, causing a serious pulmonary embolism and possibly death. If the vascular system is cared for

properly, these thrombi will not occur. Thrombophlebitis of the leg within our own family provided an
occasion to use some of the concepts developed in
the Edgar Cayce material. The physician is told to
"heal thyself." So, Gladys and I went to work on her
left great saphenous vein when it became inflamed
several years ago. There was tenderness, moderate
to severe pain, and palpable thrombus but no edema
or excessive accumulation of fluid in the tissues. As
the condition developed, inflammation appeared over
the vein as it coursed up over the medial aspect of
the knee. Some five to six inches of the structure
were clinically involved. The symptoms started one
evening, worsened during the night, and therapy
did not begin until mid-morning the next day. The
treatment we used was:

1. Light, high-vitamin diet with forced fluids.
2. Castor oil pack over the affected area, held in
   place with an Ace bandage.
3. Increased vitamin intake (probably not necessary
   if #1 is followed).
4. The healing hands of a friend.

Diet, in our opinion, is a valuable therapeutic tool
in every illness, but especially in an acute condition.
The castor oil pack has always been the most important of these treatments in these and similar cases
over the years. We have not usually had experienced
people around who can project healing from their
hands, so we have had to be content with the love
that comes with my own hands in applying care and
the castor oil pack. Since we are most commonly
working with physical applications to bring healing
of the body, we have a consciousness that responds
to such modalities most easily, and if limited to one
therapy, we would have used the castor oil pack.

The results were remarkable, as was the case in
some of our prior experiences with thrombophlebitis that were superficial. The castor oil pack was left
on during the daytime hours of the first and second
day. By the time twenty-four hours had passed, there
was no redness, no pain, and only a faint residual

tenderness. Within thirty-six hours, there were no remaining symptoms or abnormal findings; Gladys was well; and there was no recurrence.

The usual response to thrombophlebitis therapy of a conventional nature—an elastic bandage and an antiinflammatory agent—is to experience relief from pain and swelling in five to seven days. If unresolved by then, vascular surgery is often recommended. Excision of the affected veins can then hasten a cure and prevent deep extension of the thrombus and possible pulmonary embolism. Nothing is mentioned in traditional medical literature about the importance of dietary principles either in preventing or in treating a thrombophlebitis; and certainly castor oil packs have not as yet evolved into the generally accepted medical practice.

Varicose Veins

The veins of the lower extremities can get into trouble in other ways. When there is enough systemic toxicity or mechanical trauma, varicosities can develop. These usually come in the legs because the veins there undergo the greatest strain of any of the body veins, due to the upright position of the body and the gravitational force on the walls of these structures.

Childbirth sometimes causes varicosities, due to pressures from the position of the growing infant inside the uterus. But most commonly there are underlying problems (gallbladder disease, improper kidney and bladder function, general toxicity, etc.) that lay the foundation for the beginning of the varicose veins. It is usually the varicosities, in turn, that make possible thrombophlebitis. So there are many relationships within the vascular system. Therapy that we have found effective includes some of the suggestions that have already been given:

1. Improve the circulation of the lower extremities through: elastic stockings or bandages while up and about; frequent elevation of the legs when possible; massage of the legs using a stimulating

oil (equal parts of olive oil, tincture of myrrh, and compound tincture of benzoin, for instance), and walking instead of standing. Walking, Cayce said, is always the best exercise.

2. Osteopathic manipulations designed to relieve pressures on the involved nerve pathways.
3. Improve eliminations.
4. Dietary factors to bring about a better acid-alkaline balance.
5. Mullein tea.

Take internally Mullein Tea not more than 3 times a week, but make it fresh each time it is taken. Prepare a tea made from Mullein. For uniformity, preferably use the dry Mullein, a pinch between thumb and forefinger. Put into a teacup and pour boiling water on same. Let this stand for 30 minutes, strain, cool and drink. This is a reaction to the liver, the lungs, the heart and the kidneys, as to produce coordinating activity in circulation. It works with each of these and also makes a better condition through the alimentary canal.

5148–1

Paroxysmal Tachycardia

Leaving the subject of blood vessels for a bit, I would like to discuss an instance of an unusual therapy for paroxysmal tachycardia. This kind of a problem occurs when the electrical supply to the heart becomes disoriented, in a sense, and a locus of stimulation of the heartbeat sets itself up in the wall of the heart instead of allowing heart contractions to be directed by the group of nerves outside the heart that nature designed. This makes the heartbeat double or sometimes close to triple what it normally is, and often the subject will feel chest pains, making him think he is having a heart attack. It is a rather frequent condition and can in most instances be prevented or eliminated through following the suggestions already outlined in this chapter; but, to treat the immediate symptoms, a number of innovative measures have been devised by creative clinicians over the years. Sometimes these measures meet with success, sometimes without results of any kind.

Two or three years ago, a woman in her late middle years became a patient in the Clinic, and her doctor suggested a new manner of approaching the resolution of the rapid heartbeat. She was instructed to take a deep breath, then plunge her face into very cold water—just momentarily, but long enough to feel the cold. She thought this was a strange sort of procedure, and did not do it until her second or third visit after that, when she was queried about her success. The suggestion was reinforced, the face went underwater, and the tachycardia ceased immediately. It is something like holding one's breath, or breathing into a bag, or making pressure on the side of the neck. Apparently, it has a shocklike effect on the autonomic nervous system, and this breaks up the pattern of excessively rapid heartbeat.

Some Additional Comments

It is obvious that we have not dealt with a number of cardiac and vascular conditions that cause considerable disability and frequently death. The principles of prevention and of general rehabilitation or regeneration, however, apply here as well and are to be used to promote better health for the individual who chooses to use them. It is not easy, but it is usually worth the effort.

Chapter Twenty Three
BONES, JOINTS AND LIGAMENTS

When thinking of bones and joints, I immediately recall a patient who was nearing retirement age and had developed a knee that was stiff and painful. He was overweight and never ate a consistently good diet—he liked to spoil himself. While seeing me for a mildly increased blood pressure, he indicated that his knee had been giving him trouble for several months. Realizing that he was not particularly apt in following specific instructions, I suggested the simplest remedy I knew: massaging the knee with peanut oil, which could be bought at the nearest supermarket. A month later, when I saw him again, his knee was completely free of symptoms. Peanut oil massaged into the afflicted joint was one of the most common suggestions in the Cayce readings for problems such as this.

Sprains, fractures, and arthritis all need treatment by specialists in those fields when the problem is severe, but there is much that can be done before one needs to consult an orthopod and often more after the orthopod is finished. Cayce had much to say about arthritis and its therapy.

In the 1930s, Cayce specifically suggested that a naturopathic doctor seek surgical assistance at Johns Hopkins Hospital for a patient's depressed skull fracture that had not healed properly and was still causing pressure on the brain. No amount of massage or application of physical therapy would restore that area back to normal for this man. Cayce saw all treatments, however, as physical applications for healing, as he always related them to a consciousness and an awareness of God:

> Remember, applications physical—or mechanical applications, or medications or such active forces are an expression of the divine; as must be the prayers and meditations of those if they would bring help to the body.
>
> 1289-2

Fractures and sprains are given special treatment in the Edgar Cayce material based on the concept that man is essentially an electrically oriented and activated being, subject to changes through "vibratory" influences such as magnetic fields and electrically charged substances. It has already been demonstrated in laboratories all over the United States that electricity introduced into the area of a nonunited fracture of a bone will cause healing to come about where it had not previously been obtained. Cayce suggested massage in such instances with a mixture of vinegar and salt—electrolytes certainly—and experience has proved that these administrations are certainly helpful.

Some Therapies for Sprains and Fractures

I received a letter in 1976 from Frank and Dorothy Oswald, A.R.E. members in attendance at a meeting in Virginia Beach. The following is an extract from their letter:

> We heard you at the Beach a year ago last summer. My husband was the one with a broken collar bone. As soon as we arrived home we started the salt, vinegar, myrrh, olive oil treatment. The bone specialist at the next visit (a month from that time) said, "I've never seen a collar bone heal that fast in an adult."

In readings for a forty-year-old man (438–5) who was recovering from a fracture of the patella, and stiff knee ligaments as well, Cayce recommended:

> *First day* use equal parts of Olive Oil and Tincture of Myrrh as a massage.
>
> *Second day* use table salt and pure apple vinegar as a massage.
>
> Use these on alternate days; they may cause pain at first.

One of my closest friends suffered a dislocated shoulder, which was treated by his orthopedic surgeon and reduced. However, he continued to have pain and swelling in the shoulder, with fifty-percent restriction in function. He started the same course of treatment as suggested above, and gradually, over a period of several months, his shoulder returned to normal. It was not immediate, but his patience and persistence in massaging the shoulder produced a normal joint.

Here is another oil recommended by the readings to aid in the restoration of a fractured knee:

Peanut oil	4 oz.
Oil of pine needles	1 oz.
Oil of sassafras root	1 oz.
Melted lanolin	½ oz.

The substances are to be added in the order given and used as a massage, alternating the massage with salt-vinegar rubs.

These particular substances are not the only possible therapy for a sprain. I recall a woman I saw in the emergency room of the hospital some years ago. I had never seen her before. She had sprained her ankle and it was causing her a great deal of pain. X-rays indicated no fracture, so I suggested that she wrap the ankle in a castor oil pack, using an Ace bandage to hold it in place, and keep it on as much as possible over the weekend. I saw her again the first of the week, and she had neither pain nor swelling.

At an A.R.E. week-long program at Asilomar State Park in California, a fifty-five-year-old woman who was in one of my classes sprained her ankle—not severely, but painfully, and badly enough to make her limp severely through the afternoon classes and dinner. That evening, for an hour and a half, she (of her own accord) wrapped her ankle in a castor oil pack with a heating pad applied over the pack. Then, when she went to bed, she just pinned a towel around the pack after removing the heating pad. The next morning I saw her hiking around the Asilomar grounds, enjoying the scenery—no limp, no pain, and, as I found out afterward, no swelling or residual symptoms from the sprain.

From the Cayce readings, an answer to a question about weak arches demonstrated a point about healing, and about doing something yourself.

Q-18: Why have my arches always been weak? Can I ever go without wearing arch supports in my shoes?

A-18: To be sure, especially if the limbs and foot—
especially the burses in the heel, or the Achilles
burse—are stimulated. For such stimulation (besides the massage to the sacral and lumbar plex-
uses that stimulates impulses to the lower limbs),
we would advise using a compound prepared in
this manner (which will give the body a good deal
to do for itself!):

Each evening before retiring, bathe the foot and
limbs to the knees in a very mild tannic acid;
which may best be made (for such conditions) from
coffee grounds. When they are ready to be thrown
out, put on a cupful to a gallon and a half of
water. Let boil for ten minutes, pour off and allow
to cool sufficiently so that the lower limbs may be
bathed in it. Massage the limbs and the foot,
especially the heels and the arches and toes, all
the time they are in the solution, see? The whole
quantity being used, of course; drain the dregs
off, or the grounds; and keep the limbs and foot
in same for twenty minutes.

After taking them out of the solution, massage
them with *this* compound for five to ten minutes;
putting the ingredients together in the order
named:

Russian White Oil	½ pint
Witch Hazel	2 ounces
Rub Alcohol	4 ounces
Oil of Sassafras	3 minims
Tincture of Capsici	2 minims

That would make it hot enough! Massage only
the amount the skin will absorb. Shake the
solution together, for the tendency will be for
the Oil of Sassafras to rise to the top—see?
Pour a small quantity in a saucer, and only
massage into the feet and to the limbs to the
knees, including the knees. And do it yourself!
And we'll be rid of all this trouble, and it'll help
the body in many different ways. It'll walk ten
miles instead of five!

386—3

Arthritis

There are two major types of arthritis and they differ significantly—osteoarthritis (hypertrophic), which causes a buildup of calcium in the joints, tendons, and ligaments, and rheumatoid (atrophic) arthritis, which produces inflammatory changes and ultimate loss of calcium. These are lengthy and complicated problems, and thousands of physicians are dedicating their lives to the treatment and study of human beings afflicted with arthritis.

It is probably sufficient to say here that according to the Cayce readings, arthritis is generally caused by *improper eliminations*. However, the solution to this disease is not as simple as the cause; and the cause itself is not quite that simple. The severity of the illness found in rheumatoid arthritis, along with its proper prognosis, would lead one to suspect that its abnormal physiology is of a much deeper origin and possesses much more profound ramifications. At the same time, there are certain basic causal factors common to both arthritic conditions—namely, poor eliminations, with their associated and sometimes resultant condition, inadequate and imperfect assimilation. Thus, the diet that one eats and the adequacy of his eliminations through their four channels become of prime importance to successful reversal of the arthritis symptoms. Both assimilation and elimination can be influenced in many ways, and sometimes the therapy is not directly related to either of these functions, although they still have an important influence.

Let us take the case of a sixty-eight-year-old man whom I have cared for over a long period of time. He was first seen nearly ten years ago with a semirigid spine due to advanced hypertrophic arthritis. He could rotate his head right and left perhaps only five degrees either way, and his entire spine was limited drastically in all directions of movement. For one solid year, his wife used an electrically driven massager on his upper spine and neck just ten minutes each night before he went to bed. This was *every single night* without a miss. At that point he had

rotation of the head up to thirty degrees in each
direction, and could even look around over his shoulder to see if there was a car approaching from the
rear. His spine was much looser, and he was encouraged. Today, he has full rotation of his head,
having continued on a modified program. He did
alter his diet from the first, and he always had a
positive attitude about his recovery. Since the body
can absorb calcium, the function of severely calci-
fied vetebrae can indeed be restored. All this did not
happen because of the local effects derived from the
daily massage by his wife. There was nevertheless a
considerable influence on the organs of assimilation—
the stomach, pancreas, liver, gallbladder, etc.—because of the neurological activity induced by the
massage to the sympathetic ganglia in the upper
dorsal area of the spine. So help comes in many
ways!

Diet for the arthritis patient assumes a major role
as he starts a program of therapy recommended by
the readings. It always seemed that the diet should
be of a laxative nature. Over and over, Cayce advised
that celery, lettuce, carrots, and watercress be used
frequently together with gelatin as a salad. This, he
said, would enhance the values found in all these
vegetables and in the gelatin itself, and would be
beneficial to the body. For some individuals, figs
and dates were suggested to provide the laxative
effect, and vegetable juices were found to be especially helpful. Cooked beets and carrots, and vegetables of all kinds, in large measure were always in
order; while one meal of green raw vegetables at
noon was frequently suggested.

Fish, fowl, and lamb were seen as the primary
source of meat; and no fried foods were to be
permitted. It is questionable whether any person
with arthritis should ever use much salt (sodium
chloride type). Starches and sweets together should
also be avoided; and this means no cakes and
pastries. Honey or corn syrup or buckwheat cakes or
corn bread or the like would be all right, but not
together with white bread. Apparently, the white
flour that is used in cakes, pastries, and bread,

when combined with sweets, yields detrimental effects. The diet should be well balanced but should contain no starchy foods. Green leafy vegetables are always excellent, and they should be used in preference to the pod or bulbar type. Wild game is also excellent food for the arthritic. A frequent dietary theme from the readings is to increase raw vegetables, decrease meats, allow no carbonated drinks, alcohol, or stimulants, and avoid fats: alkalinity produced from such a diet seems to be the goal.

To increase eliminations, various approaches are helpful: castor oil packs, five or six drops of castor oil, orally, nightly before retiring, colonics, or enemas. Hydrotherapy in a variety of forms is helpful: ordinary hot baths, Epsom salts baths (two and a half to five or even ten pounds of Epsom salts in a full tub of water, soaking the body for five or ten minutes or longer—until a good sweat develops), fume baths, steam-cabinet treatments, Jacuzzi or hot tub or sitz baths. Massage, treatments with an electric vibrator massager, or osteopathic treatments are important means of increasing lymphatic drainage and loosening up the muscles and tendons. Exercise also performs these functions. Oils are frequently used with the massages; particularly effective are olive oil and peanut oil, two ounces each, with one ounce of lanolin. For case 3244, who apparently had a great problem with his assimilations, Cayce recommended the following combination of oils:

Usoline or Nujol (Russian White Oil)	4 oz.
Oil of pine needles	1 oz.
Olive oil	1 oz.
Peanut oil	1 oz.
Lanolin, liquified	1 oz.

Another combination of oils was given in the readings to be used only after an Epsom salts bath—bringing about a degree of heat and irritation, which is actually preferable at times:

Usoline or Nujol	4 oz.
Peanut oil	2 oz.

Sassafras root oil	½ oz.
Oil of pine needles	½ oz.
Oil of mustard	¼ oz.

In the readings, Atomidine was suggested to be taken internally in nearly every case of arthritis. It was given in numerous cycles—and always in cycles (see Circulating File on Arthritis). Our most common prescription to patients has been to take one drop on Monday, two on Tuesday, three on Wednesday, and so on up to Friday (five drops); then discontinue over the weekend and start all over again with one drop the first of the next week. This procedure would be followed the first three weeks of each month.

People who correspond with us, however, rarely follow just that prescribed course of treatment. One woman, who was a long-time arthritis sufferer, wrote that she was not taking any medication for her arthritis, even though she had been afflicted with it for ten years. This is her story:

> I recently started drinking olive oil. I took approximately six tablespoons a day (during the day) for two weeks, then I took one tablespoon a day for two weeks. The pain in every joint was gone. I stopped this procedure, feeling maybe the arthritis may have been arrested, as some cases do.
>
> After three weeks, the pain started to return. I knew it must be the olive oil, so I started taking three tablespoons a day for one week, then discontinuing dosage. After two weeks, the pain was only slight but returning. I took only three tablespoons just one day a week. All I take now is three tablespoons for one day, and it lasts one week and no pain for this period.

This kind of therapy was never suggested in the readings, and it appears that the woman was, in fact, just holding down the symptoms, but not really reversing the root causes. However, two more stories about oils and their usefulness in arthritis bear telling.

In reading Jess Stearn's *Edgar Cayce*, I noted with much interest his references to arthritis and the use of pure peanut oil. As a rheumatoid arthritic I have found it to be of great benefit to my condition. After using peanut oil as a massaging oil for several years, I have to agree with Cayce's belief that it not only lubricates but heals as well. I am sure that had I known about the oil in this use I would have been spared much misery. Why isn't the use of peanut oil to reduce joint inflammation and pain in arthritis better known? Does the medical profession spurn it as a home remedy?

And from California:

Mother had arthritis so bad she was committed to the hospital. She was there for two weeks and released with no apparent help. The arthritis was centered in her fingers which were doubled back in her palms—she didn't think she would be able to open up her fingers again. Father brought her home and started a treatment of hot castor oil—rubbing her hands, arms, and shoulders and legs three times a day. Within a period of three or four months her condition improved to the extent she could walk, use her arms, and her hands straightened out and today she is completely cured. She was seventy-six years old when she was at her worst and is now eighty-one.

Chapter Twenty Four
THE EYES AND EARS
—THE SENSES

In the Edgar Cayce readings, there are three nervous systems described, not the usual two. There is the cerebrospinal nervous system, designed in man to control conscious action and muscular movement: it is the functional component in the body of man for the conscious mind. Second is the sympathetic nervous system, or what we recognize today as the autonomic nervous system. In the days when Cayce gave his information, the autonomic was, for a period, called the sympathetic or vegetative. The autonomic is the nervous system for the unconscious mind. The third system is the sensory nervous system; functionally the only means by which we can be aware that we are living in a three-dimensional world. This latter system involves all the nerves that supply the five senses and is closely intertwined and involved with the other two systems of neural transmission.

One of the interesting concepts coming out of this triune neural model is that sense perceptions (color, for instance) are really communicated to the autonomic nervous system before they are registered consciously in the brain. This primary connection may provide us with some understanding as to why our appetites are increased by the rich brown colors or reds or oranges of one restaurant, while the unwary owner of another eating establishment down the street loses customers because his restaurant is painted in blues and whites.

We also recognize the reality of this close neural relationship when we become aware that the smell of a certain perfume takes us unerringly back to a specific time and place and person; or perhaps the gentle strains of a song heard once again recall a distant, warm, meaningful experience. And from the popular comic strip "Peanuts" comes Linus clutching his blanket so closely: he feels it and appears to remember something unconsciously.

It might easily be said that the sensory nervous system *is* the autonomic, or at least a part of it; and, in reality, we do function as a whole person, with all our parts making up one individual. However, if we are to continue to perceive each human being as an ongoing entity, a spiritual being, having an origin and a destiny in a spiritual realm that we only faintly discern, then it becomes reasonable to look at the body as a means created for us to experience this world. Our unconscious minds move us most of the time, even though we are often unaware of the body's movements or of the mind's control. The mind, furthermore, may be projected not only as an unconscious reality, but as a conscious mind that deals with our Earthly dimension. It is the sensory nervous system that provides the means for communicating with this world.

It is through our sensory apparatus that we stimulate memories and touch on habit patterns that are part of all we have done and felt and seen and tasted and smelled and heard perhaps throughout the ages of our recurrent lifetimes on Earth.

The sensory nervous system was to Mr. Cayce a unit that enabled man to become aware of his external environment. Such a relationship is further underscored by the following story. Carter C. Collins, a professor of biophysics at the Pacific School of Medical Sciences, reported some years ago that he had developed a tiny, spectacle-mounted television camera that enables a blind man to see by relaying pictures through nerve endings in the skin of the abdomen, and, after a period of training, the information from the skin reaches the centers of consciousness as a visual image and not in the sense of touching something.

There is also the story of an experiment done with one-celled creatures (somewhat like the well-known paramecium) called tetrahymena pyriformis. They have a specific avoidance reaction that makes them stop, back up, and take off in a different direction every time they meet an obstacle. A very small electrical source was introduced into the tank of water. When the electricity was introduced, the tetrahymena stopped, backed up, and took off in a different direction. A strong searchlight was directed at the tank. When the light was turned on by itself without the electricity, there was no response by the tetrahymena. Then, electricity and light were turned on at the same time seventeen or eighteen times consecutively. The avoidance reaction occurred each time. Then, the next time, the light was turned on without the electricity. The tetrahymena stopped, backed up, and took off in a different direction. The point of this story is not only that one-celled creatures can be taught (e.g., that they have consciousness), but that there is perception of light and of painful stimuli (feeling) through the mechanism of a single cell, which has no nervous system, no sensory organs, no apparent means to support this consciousness. If one-celled creatures can do all this, and if a blind man can see through the cells of his abdomen, it means that there is indeed much to learn about man as an entity experiencing the Earth through his senses.

Cayce described some of the interrelationships among the senses, the organic functioning of the body, and the emotions, which work through the glands and their hormones. He indicated that emotions, as psychological conditions, create pathology in the organs supplied by the autonomic nervous system and in the senses themselves. To a woman describing her condition, he said:

> The emotions are the psychological conditions, the effects are to the liver, spleen, heart and sensory system—that are the present pathological conditions.
>
> 2452-1

Color Blindness

While genetic conditions are generally regarded to be incurable, this is not the case if one considers the premises of the Cayce readings that healing is always a possibility and that the body as the product of mind and spirit always possesses unlimited possibilities. Consider color blindness. In the Cayce concept of things, color blindness begins as nerve energies in the vagus nerve become deflected from their origin in the second, third, and fourth dorsal sympathetic ganglia. Normally, these nerve impulses are coordinated through the vagus nerve with similar areas of neural control existing in the third, fourth, and fifth cervical ganglia. These latter ganglia are the optic centers that control various functions of the eyes. Thus, the nerve energies that should be flowing to the optic centers have been deflected because of disturbances in the upper dorsal area, and the optic centers are thus deficient in circulatory control energy that might in turn be directed toward the eye. A complicated series of events then takes place. Swelling, reddening, and irritation then come to the eyelid, portions of the eyeball, "and to the character of that which is reflected in the lens, iris, and in the response to the optic center itself." (820–2)

Therapy for color blindness according to the Cayce readings is written up in one of the circulating files at A.R.E. Headquarters in Virginia Beach and involves: diet, osteopathic treatments (to the dorsal first, then to the cervical area), and violet ray treatments and wet cell battery treatments given in three-week cycles. Color blindness is not a frequent occurrence—only one reading was given on that condition out of the thousands Cayce originated on a variety of subjects. But the eyes and ears have much more common problems.

Inflammation of the Eye

A stye or a hordeolum is a bacterial infection and inflammation of connective tissue of the eyelid near a hair follicle. It can be external or deep, the latter being the most troublesome. We don't see such problems often in the office because they usually are cared for at home without medical advice. Somewhere in the readings I must have read about using potato poultices to the eyelid for styes, but there is currently no circulating file on this disease. However, there is an extensive file on blepharitis or inflammation of the eyelid. Probably seventy-five percent of the readings on blepharitis suggest the use of a potato poultice. We have used this particular old-time therapy in a number of cases of stye and have found it to be extremely effective, clearing up the average inflammation in twenty-four to thirty-six hours and often after just one application of the poultice.

Cayce suggested that eliminations were a problem in most cases where blepharitis occurred, so he usually suggested that eliminations be improved as he recommended the use of the poultices. The poultice, he said, would in a sense draw off inflammation. It was important to use the old Irish potato, not the new, and it was used sometimes wrapped in a thin gauze cloth and sometimes directly upon the closed eyelid. This is one of the old-time simple remedies that works like a charm on a variety of problems about the eye. Perhaps it has something to do with the enzymes that are released when the potato is scraped down into a mushlike poultice. I also suspect that it has a beneficial effect on the entire eyeball, most probably improving the lymphatic drainage, thus cleansing the tissues and making them more functional.

Cataracts

Cataracts of the eye are common in eighty-year-old women, although eighty-year-olds are not so common. Sometimes, at the A.R.E. Clinic, we find it to be very important to treat a person where they are in consciousness, in a sense improvising from our own experience what we think needs to be done. By utilizing our knowledge of physiology, we come to a conclusion as to what specific therapy should be used.

One elderly patient, seeking to improve her physical body without undergoing the difficulties of surgery, wanted to use something that she could apply herself, since she lived alone. She was told to use potato poultices on her eyes twice a week. She was also using the head and neck exercises, which are beneficial to do in all conditions of the senses, and she was given Glycothymoline packs for her sinuses, which had caused her some trouble.

She followed our directions to the letter, and was very persistent, consistent, and patient in her approach. Eye examinations about a year and three months later revealed that the cataracts were still there but had not progressed, while her vision had improved. Her letter of the same date tells the story better:

I have an appointment with you, in about two months, but I couldn't wait to tell you the good news—I'm back to wearing my glasses again—they seem to be almost perfect! Now, I can read with BOTH eyes, instead of one. I had abandoned them about a year and a half ago, as I had so much trouble focusing with them, and after taking your treatments with the grated raw potato, and the Glycothymoline compresses, my sight seemed to improve enough, so I could carry on. I realized they were getting better and better, but did not think to try my glasses until last Sunday. Of course, this gives me much more confidence in driving, which I had been somewhat reluctant about, especially on the crowded highways. I am praising God and blessing you. . . .

Other Eye Conditions

So-called granulated eyelids are responsive to a treatment of bathing in a weak solution of boric acid and then using the potato poultice twice a week in the evening before retiring. We have found that these poultices are frequently helpful in most conditions of the eye, but there are other suggested remedies in the Cayce readings.

For conjunctivitis, an eye bath solution of Glycothymoline one part and distilled water two parts can be used. This is a stronger solution than Cayce suggested in another reading, where the amounts were two tablespoons of the Glycothymoline to one quart of water. No doubt some individuals are more sensitive to substances such as Glycothymoline than others.

Dr. Mayo Hotten reported to me on a small series of cases where he treated pterygium of the eye using castor oil packs and reduced the inflammation sufficiently to perhaps "prevent surgery." From another correspondent, a report came to us about the successful use of castor oil on a stye of the lower eyelid. Usually these recurrent styes need incision and drainage.

Lee Sannella, a cooperating doctor in the Edgar

Cayce Foundation program, is a psychiatrist and specialist in opthalmology. Some of his recent work has come to the attention of those working in the field of biofeedback training. A report in *Behavior Today* tells of his work with glaucoma. Using techniques that included Bates exercises, reflexology techniques, autogenic training, self-rhythmization exercises, alpha/theta monitoring, and some other methods, Lee reported that five of six persons suffering from glaucoma were successful in lowering eye pressure during a one-day workshop. His comments on this work are as interesting as his results:

> There seems to be an essential factor of consent and agreement in healing—a consent or affirmation that the patient really wants to be free of the condition, and an agreement that the formatory, everyday functional level shall be set aside or bypassed in favor of contacting a deeper level of body physiology. . . . Once the body is given a chance to start regularizing or healing, the tendency spreads.

The Sannella work reminds me of the many readings in which Cayce pointed out the importance of the mind as a builder, and the source of all healing as coming from Creative Spirit or God.

Hearing Impairments

The problems of the ear and the hearing itself are probably not as numerous as those involving the eye but can be quite as distressing. When one looks at deafness from the wider viewpoint, physical disturbances appear as immediate apparent causes; however, psychological and spiritual factors are involved in the background as basic causes. Modern psychiatry recognizes that hearing problems in the older person often are caused by that person's becoming "tired" of listening to others, and developing an actual physical condition because of this emotional reaction. Deafness has often been described in the Cayce life readings as a karmic thing—a result of one's turning a "deaf ear" to someone else's needs at a critical time in a past life.

Whatever the cause from an immutable past, there are the physical conditions that have developed to create deafness in those who are to any extent physically deaf. Cayce recognized this as he gave physical readings, and, in a typical remark from the unconscious state, he gave the following information about a thirty-five-year-old woman who had suddenly lost her hearing:

> As we find, there are disturbing conditions and these primarily began from a catarrhal condition in the nasal passages and in the throat. These effects upon the body cause a great deal of acidity, and the lack of eliminations causes the suppression of supplying of the flow of energies to the organs of the sensory system.
>
> 5315–1

In making recommendations for a number of people, Cayce suggested several therapeutic approaches, which included osteopathy or mechanotherapy to the cervical area, finger surgery to the eustachian tube area, cleansing of the intestinal tract, wet-cell-battery treatment, general buildup of the body, head and neck exercises, and several other modalities at various times.

Recent activities in the field of hearing defects include some very fascinating work done by researchers at the Cleveland Hearing and Speech Center in Ohio. There, a headphonelike unit broadcasts a low-frequency radio signal to the auditory nerves, which are thus stimulated and reactivated—at least to a degree. Dr. Jenkins-Lee, who heads the work, likens the inner ear to an electrical-chemical complex, much like the battery of a car (indeed, all cells of the body are actually galvanic electrical units), and the device, in a sense, recharges the hearing apparatus, bringing about an improvement in hearing.

Chinese doctors visit children at a special colony and treat them daily with simple but effective acupuncture. All the children are among those we call "deaf and dumb," when the treatments begin. But they begin to hear and talk and are taught to sing to improve their voices. It is known that the sounds from the outside world coming into the brain create the necessary pathways for a child learning to speak. If sound is kept out beyond two or three years of age, due to hearing loss of any kind, then the speech of that child will be either absent or abnormal. Recent work by Dr. Philip Peltzman under the sponsorship of the Telephone Pioneers of America has utilized the computer and the electroencephalogram to determine whether there is a hearing loss in a newborn infant. Then, measures can be brought about to aid the child in hearing, and much grief and difficult life experiences can be avoided. These examples remind us that changes of an apparently irreversible nature can be corrected, at least partially; and that it is really the functional components of the human body that we should be working on and working with.

Hearing loss in a very young person is a highly disturbing thing to parents, and sometimes makes a doctor wish he had taken up another profession, the responses to therapy usually being so slow and so difficult to come by. One case that we can draw upon demonstrates some of the concepts of physiological rehabilitation about which we have been talking. Jill was born in February 1968 and came under our care when she was two years old, with complaints of loose stools and some vomiting. In June 1970, her mother reported that Jill was having trouble with her hearing yet apparently had not had much in the way of ear infections. Triaminic syrup had been used unsuccessfully. In November she was seen with a left otitis media or inflammation of the ear and was treated with an analgesic ear drop and antibiotic orally. There were also symptoms of upper respiratory infection, and the tonsils were greatly enlarged or hypertrophic. She continued through the winter having some troubles and was seen in January 1971 by an ear specialist (otologist), primarily for her diminished hearing. He reported:

Examination revealed dull ear drums bilaterally and a diagnosis of hypertrophied adenoids with bilateral serous otitis media was made. I advised that an adenoidectomy be performed and bilateral myringotomies and that tubes be inserted. The child has been scheduled for this surgery February 23 at St. Joseph's Hospital.

The mother did not really want any surgery done and so declined the surgical procedure. I saw the child in mid-February, at which time her tonsils were still enlarged, the ears appeared normal, her breathing was normal, and the mother stated that she thought Jill was hearing better. She was given small doses of Atomidine for several weeks and was well until March, when she developed a repeat left otitis media. She responded well to an antibiotic again, but her hearing became gradually and noticeably worse, which brought her again to our office in late June. I scheduled her for an audiometric exam at Good Samaritan Hospital. This was reported by the department director as follows:

In summary, the pure tone data indicate that your patient's hearing in the right ear is within the lower limits of normalcy, whereas she sustains a mild loss in the left ear with a significant conductive component which, perhaps, is bilateral. The test results were discussed with the informant, and it was suggested that the patient return to you with regards to the conductive impairment.

Jill's mother reported to the examiner at this point that Jill's hearing problem had been a constant thing for a period of two years, so it is obvious that it had never really cleared up—at least in her mother's estimation. Therapy was started in late June with head and neck exercises as Cayce had so often described them; the Atomidine was started again with a half drop in half a glass of water each morning five days a week; and, several days later, she began the use of an inhalant, five deep breaths at a treatment, three treatments a day. The inhalant was made up of the following ingredients:

Grain alcohol	4 ounces
Oil of eucalyptus	20 minims
Canadian balsam	5 minims
Guiacol benzoate	5 minims
Rectified creosote	3 minims
Tincture benzoin	10 minims
Rectified oil turpentine	5 minims
Tincture tolu balsam	30 minims

Jill's mother reported in the beginning of July that she felt certain the hearing was improved, so a repeat audiogram was scheduled for August 18. The graph from this report gave evidence that Jill was now hearing normally. Her mother was instructed to keep up the same therapy program for another six weeks before discontinuing and checking again at the Clinic.

A theory of what happened might go like this: through the use of the head and neck exercises affecting the spine, spinal cord, recurrent branches of the spinal nerves, sympathetic ganglia, and the circulatory and sensory centers that are found in that area, the nerve and circulatory supply to the sensory apparatus is improved. Cayce suggests in his readings that the Atomidine, even in such minute amounts, stimulates the glandular cells of the body to a better response as they attempt to "do their thing." And what does the inhalant accomplish? Through the tissues and cells of the entire upper respiratory tract, nasal passages, adenoids, tonsils, sinuses, and eustachian tubes, there is a cleansing that comes about.

Perhaps—with the proper incentive, the proper simple assistance, the proper attitudes, the proper diet—the body can indeed rehabilitate itself, bring itself to a state of balance and homeostasis that we call healing.

Music Therapy

We cannot leave the subject of the senses without touching on some of the effects of music when music is used as therapy. Emotions are certainly quieted down or aroused by a variety of musical compositions—one type soothes us or lulls us to sleep, while another stirs our martial instincts or our basic drives and urges.

Several years ago it came to my attention that one French researcher is playing the works of the masters through a device that influences cell tissue by transforming sounds into direct vibrations. The patient listens while the tunes are further relayed through electrodes attached to the body. Meanwhile, an Italian physician has been using Bach fugues to treat indigestion, and it has been found that Mozart is an ideal choice when working with rheumatism. Beethoven is considered good for hernias, while Handel helps "broken hearts" and other disturbed emotional states. For insomnia?—try Schubert.

We discussed in this chapter how psychological disturbances work through the endocrine glands and their hormones to produce illness in the body and the senses. Similarly, if music is creative in nature and the effect is purely psychological, then it is reasonable to anticipate that hormonal benefit in the body can be experienced and illnesses can be corrected.

In a program for a limited number of patients at the Clinic, we use music as a bridge between the conscious and the unconscious minds. When high-quality music is played at a higher than normal intensity, and combined with a massage of the body tissues done in rhythm with the music, memories and subconscious disturbances are brought up from the information stored in the unconscious mind, sometimes in the very cells of the body, where memory also exists. People recall past lives this way, and recall relationships in this and prior lives that can be dealt with constructively in a helpful environment. We call this the Temple Beautiful Program, lasting seventeen days and incorporating many other modalities into a treatment plan.

Other Therapies

Auriculotherapy is a method of using acupuncture on the ear, and thereby influencing functions throughout the body. Some physicians use only this method of treatment, disregarding all others. In chapter 11, I described an exercise of the ear that may be helpful for the hearing, much like the Chinese exercise for the eyes is helping people throughout China to maintain better eyesight. It has a major difference in that the entire body is influenced by the exercise, as well as just the ear. How much it might help can only be demonstrated by use, for its action is through neural impulses that cannot be traced adequately nor measured.

A story about tinnitus or sounding in the ears and dizziness was volunteered by one of my patients who had been bothered with this condition for some time. He had not been troubled by wax in the ears, which will often cause such symptoms. Knowing the variety of ways in which castor oil can be used, this patient decided to use some castor oil drops in his ears. He continued regularly for a period of about two months, and his dizziness completely left and most of his ringing was gone.

From another correspondent I learned that her mother had started to do the head and neck exercises along with some breathing exercises, and "after *extreme* drainage, her hearing is practically normal where once we had to almost shout to make ourselves heard."

The earlobe also benefits from castor oil, but here it must be given locally. One long-time A.R.E. member relates her experience with castor oil together with that of her sister:

> . . . Four years ago . . . I had my ears pierced. They became infected and stayed that way for some time. I spent a small fortune on doctors and medicine. I finally remembered the castor oil and used it several times a day—and in three days' time my ears were completely healed and I've had no trouble since then.

But then she goes on with her story:

> My sister also used warmed castor oil drops in her ears after doctors told her her hearing had been impaired by having a shotgun go off close to her. She had a fifty percent hearing loss and a loud ringing. Since using the castor oil drops her hearing has improved and the ringing has almost stopped. I am looking forward to a long association with A.R.E.

No wonder!

Good Sense Therapy

It is implied in the Cayce readings that all the senses gain improvement through proper use of diet, by using the head and neck exercises regularly, probably by use of osteopathic or chiropractic treatments, and by an emotional-attitudinal direction in life that is accepting in its nature. For the senses can be shut off if we reject what our Earth experience is trying to teach us, and the senses are the only means we have as spiritual beings to relate to those lessons. So it would benefit us to accept what life has to offer us—it will help keep us alert in our sensorium during the days and years we spend here.

Chapter Twenty Five
PROBLEMS UNIQUE TO WOMEN

Ovulation, conception, and childbearing are subjects close to everyone. Medicine, religion, and science have specific points of view on how each of these activities comes about; and the Edgar Cayce readings also add some interesting insights.

Ovulation is an act of nature and has its own little cycles and peculiarities that depend on a variety of factors. Conception is another matter: when the sperm penetrates the egg or ovum, conception takes place, for the two cells become one and the process of cell division begins, bringing into being a whole new physical body. While conception is considered an act of nature, no one seems to take into account the fact that penetration by one sperm out of potentially thousands involves a specific electrical phenomenon. Every cell membrane is part of a cellular electrical unit. In the Cayce readings, it is repeatedly suggested that electricity is a manifestation of the Creative Force, or God. This underscores the statement by Cayce that conception is "an act of God."

Interestingly, both science and religion state that there are those rare occasions when birth can occur without the intervention of the sperm. Scientific investigators have discovered this phenomenon among turkeys, where such immaculate conception always produces a male. Similarly, the Catholic Church accepts that not only was Jesus immaculately conceived by Mary, but that Mary herself was immaculately conceived by her mother, Anne. It is interesting to note that the Edgar Cayce readings agree with both of these postulates. Cayce saw conception as an act of God as well as that which we as human beings have as our destiny:

> . . . Souls will evolve into the manner to be able to bring into the world souls, even as Mary did. And these may come as souls of men and women become more and more aware that these channels, these temples of the body are *indeed* the temple of the living God and may be used for those communications with God, the Father of the souls of men!

> 1158–5

Stress

Following conception are the nine months of pregnancy. During that time, stresses occur. Sometimes these stresses are compensated for, and at other times they cause damage. There are also other influences on the unborn child that have not been well understood—influences that relate to what the mother thinks and feels, and what the father chooses as his attitude during this period.

It has long been noted that anxiety-prone mothers give birth to infants of lower birthweights. Folklore suggests that a pregnant woman might "lose her baby" if she is subjected to fright or great anxiety. Maternal stress in pregnancy and its effect upon the health and vitality of the infant being carried have been studied in various research situations. Adamsons (*Contemporary OB/GYN* vol. 5, January 1975) reports on some of his work that helps clarify mechanisms by which stress has its effect on the baby. Adamsons points toward the autonomic nervous system as carrying the messages that direct these stresses, and he has shown how real they are in primates (monkeys). While monkeys are admittedly not people, the reduction in uterine blood flow and the increased uterine excitability in the monkey can readily be understood to be relevant to such circumstances in the human.

It would appear that the intrinsic anxiety with which many women approach pregnancy has not as yet been suffficiently correlated with the kinds of physiological changes familiar to the physician. Thus, the state of mind is frequently neglected even while it physiological effects are being noted in the pregnant woman and in her infant. Adamsons notes that there may be a large number of patients whose babies' brain damage may have nothing to do with genetic factors or with the management of labor and delivery; but rather may be due to the attitude of mind, to the emotions, or to the altered state of the mother's sympathetic nervous system. It might even be said that a large number of all newborn infant abnormalities could be avoided by taking preventive action to relieve stress and deep emotional strain in the pregnant mother.

It has always been fascinating to see how Edgar Cayce handled concepts and stated them clearly long before modern methodology could formulate supporting scientific evidence. So far, medicine has not yet recognized that even the father's state of mind can affect the infant. Cayce said it does. Moreover, he pointed to the mother's mental and physical condition and related it to what we are as human beings from the very beginning.

> While as an individual entity, [457] presents the fact of a body, a mind, a soul—it has been given as a promise, as an opportunity to man through coition, to furnish, to create a channel through which the Creator, God, may give to individuals the opportunity of seeing, experiencing His handiwork.
>
> Then, know the attitude of mind, of self, of the companion, in creating the opportunity; for it depends upon the state of attitude as to the nature, the character that may be brought into material experience.
>
> Leave then the spiritual aspects to God. Prepare the mental and the physical body, according to the nature, the character of that soul being sought.
> 457—10

It hardly needs to be stated that anxiety and stress cannot coexist with love and affection; with the attitudes that bring about a well-balanced life and contentment in well-doing. Perhaps what is needed in obstetrics is the teaching of those qualities that Cayce often recommended, which are spoken of in the Bible as "fruits of the spirit." When these are learned, the level of anxiety goes down and the health of the unborn infant rises. Conversely, when the fruits of the spirit are not part of the ongoing experience of the new mother and her environment, complications arise.

One of the most interesting concepts I have found in the Cayce material, and one that has not yet been thoroughly studied, is the idea of using a castor oil pack on the abdomen throughout pregnancy—taken in cycles, of course. We have seen several women do this, and the child has been a healthy offspring; however, one might argue that they might well have

turned up healthy anyway. When there is a threatened abortion, we always have the mother put a
castor oil pack on her tummy. Frequently the bleeding stops and abortion is prevented. From our knowledge of how these castor oil packs do their physiological work, it seems logical to make certain assump-
tions: that the lymphatic flow in the abdomen and
particularly the uterus improves, and the cells are
thereby rendered healthier; that the autonomic nervous system becomes better balanced in its function;
and that the sense of relaxation often described makes
the entire bodily circulation more effective, aiding
both mother and baby.

Vaginal Warts

One complication of pregnancy that proves to be
very bothersome to the patient and to the physician
is the condition known as vaginal warts. Not common two decades ago, it has become a frequent
offender. One patient under our care at the A.R.E.
Clinic was found to have clusters of cauliflowerlike
vaginal warts on the external genitalia, on the wall
of the vagina surrounding the cervix, and on the
cervix itself when she was first seen at fifteen weeks
of gestation. She was treated over the next five weeks
with podophyllin locally, and the warts on the external genitalia become somewhat smaller. The vaginal
and cervical warts, however, did not respond. It was
not thought advisable to continue this treatment after
this point, but instead the patient was advised to use
gentle vaginal douches using first one tablespoon of
Glycothymoline and the next time ten drops of Atomidine, both times as an additive to a quart of water.

Subsequent visits over the next twelve weeks revealed a gradual disappearance of the warts until,
four weeks prior to her due date, the lesions were
completely gone. It is perhaps difficult to say which
therapy was most effective, or whether the recovery
was spontaneous. More importantly, the patient did
deliver spontaneously, avoiding with the disappearance of the warts what would have had to be a
Caesarean section.

Tumors

From England comes a case study that brings us back again to that ancient remedy from the plant *Racinus communis,* known more popularly as the Palma Christi, or castor oil. Carroll Yap, a cooperating physician, tells of her patient who had a uterine fibroid that increased over a five-year period to the size of an orange. A first pregnancy in 1971 ended in a still-birth. A second pregnancy was delivered by Caesarean section. The fibroid was seen protruding into the uterine cavity during the surgical procedure, so the patient was scheduled for a myectomy three months later. However, before allowing the surgery to proceed, Dr. Yap wanted to be sure about the size of the fibroid. Thus, an examination under anesthesia was to be done three months after the baby's birth. Six weeks prior to this examination, Dr. Yap started the patient on castor oil packs over the abdominal area regularly, three times a week. When the exam revealed only a questionable bulge on deep palpation or touch, and curettage or surgical scraping showed no sign of uterine tumor, the myectomy was, of course, canceled.

A forty-six-year-old female, first seen in the Clinic on November 3, 1970, had a complaint of pain in her right upper quadrant that had been present for approximately sixteen years, and that had started after she had been through a bad spell with peritonitis or inflammation of the membrane lining the abdominal wall. Her findings were: tenderness at McBurney's point with no rigidity; thickened left labia minora; uterus enlarged, with a myoma or tumor the size of a hen's egg on her right fundus; chronic phlebitis or inflammation of a vein in her left leg.

She was placed on a rehabilitative program of (1) castor oil packs over lower abdomen three times a week (three days in succession); (2) head and neck exercises daily; and (3) light massage with a Cayce oil combination to the left leg each night before retiring. Three months later, pelvic examination no longer revealed any evidence of a fibroid; the uterus

was normal in size and nontender; the abdomen
was no longer giving the patient any trouble and
was also nontender; the labia had not changed;
and the left leg had improved somewhat with the
use of the massage. The woman had been extremely
persistent in keeping up with the treatments as
directed.

A cooperating surgeon in Pennsylvania wrote me
about another unusual case.

I had a patient upon whom I performed a vaginal
hysterectomy and vaginal plastic repair. She developed a febrile post-operative course which turned
out to be due to a large pelvic abscess. On treatment with antibiotics and proteolytic enzymes,
she improved somewhat, but she had a persistent
mass about 10 × 10 cm in size which was very
tender. I wanted to perform further surgery upon
her, but she refused. For several weeks I followed
her, and her condition did not improve. She had
malaise, fever, and low abdominal pain, and her
tender pelvic mass persisted.

She still would not accept surgery, so I suggested
that she try castor oil packs daily along with the
medicine. I next saw her a month later. Although
she still had some discomfort, she was happy to
report considerable improvement. She commented:
"The packs always put me to sleep and make me
feel good all over." My examination disclosed almost complete resolution of the pelvic abscess.
There was only a small area of induration remaining in the area of the vaginal cuff which was
slightly tender. I was very surprised and pleased
with this result, and told her that I didn't feel
surgery would be necessary.

This patient also commented that she thought
flannel and castor oil was considerably less expen-
sive than having another operation.

Cystic Mastitis

Cystic mastitis causes considerable discomfort and frequently is a painful condition. The chronic irritation of the cysts formed from the glands of the breast that produce milk has been known to persist for many years. It was an unusual forty-one-year-old woman who came to the Clinic several years ago complaining of having had trouble with her breasts for six years. The case was unusual because for the last two of those six years she had been nursing her youngest child. Actually, he had been off the breast for six months, but ever since then she had had twinges of pain, which her previous doctor felt was related to the cysts. In consulting with us, she felt she would like to use the concepts of therapy found in the Cayce material, so we suggested alternating massages of the breast—not a deep massage but a gentle, firm massage—in a circular manner starting at the nipple and working out toward the outer aspect of the breast, lasting approximately five minutes. One night, she would use cocoa butter, the next night, Iodex ointment. After one week of this kind of therapy, the pain disappeared and has not recurred, even during the menstrual period. To quote the patient, she thinks the cysts have decreased in size,

> but it may be just wishful thinking. I have also had group prayers and have prayed myself. Also, I have resumed jogging (at least a mile a day). Just thought you might like to know the additional factors. Be that as it may—the modes may be various, but the source of healing is always God.

Vaginitis

Vaginitis is one of the most common problems facing the female patient. In our experience, most of these infections will respond to a series of douches—one time using a tablespoon of Glycothymoline to a quart of water, and then two days later using a teaspoon of Atomidine to a quart of water. It's best to douche at night, and to continue the alternate treatments for at least two weeks. On occasion, we will recommend the use of castor oil packs over the abdomen and osteopathic treatments to the low back. Furthermore, a basic diet insures that assimilation of the body is all right and that the probability of vaginitis recurring decreases.

In my correspondence several years ago with Dr. Ernie Poole, he had written me enthusiastically about the use of Glycothymoline douches (and no Atomidine) in treating vaginitis. Later on, he updated me on his procedures, expanding on how he has found it helpful:

> I have found, thanks to a patient's suggestion, that saturating a Tampax with Glycothymoline and applying it in this manner has given the best and most sustained results. Usually I have them use a saturated Tampax q.a.m. and h.s. for two weeks; then discontinue and see how it goes.* If recurrence is met with (although I haven't seen many) I'd simply repeat. The initial period of two weeks is not followed by many, since the symptoms abate and there is no need for prolonged use.

About the same time, I received a letter from retired physician Theodore Maday, recounting some of his time-honored uses of Epsom salts, some of them being directed at the vagina. His letter rekindled my amazement at the wide variety of therapies available to the human being to care for his illnesses. Cayce pointed this out by inference over and over again as he suggested multiple methods of approaching the satisfactory resolution to almost any problem. Individual medications or treatments were used in the Cayce readings in a variety of ways. When I researched castor oil in the Cayce material, I stopped counting after I had uncovered over fifty uses for which he had suggested it.

Problems unique to the female essentially involve disturbances of the pelvic organs and the breast.

*Q.a.m. means every morning; h.s. means at bedtime.

Those that we have covered in this chapter are typical, common problems, with typical therapeutic approaches taken from the Cayce material. There are additional treatment programs outlined in the Cayce readings for the more serious illnesses in the breast and pelvis, but they require more space than can be provided here.

Chapter Twenty Six
CHILDREN'S PROBLEMS

Gladys and I have had six children, the youngest of whom, David, is now twenty-three. While none of them qualifies as a child any longer, I can well remember when David was just a couple of years old; he was a veritable dynamo of energy. If you have ever tried to follow a child like that around for even part of a day, you will realize that it is virtually impossible. The very essence of that "life busting out" in kids may also be a part of the reason why they become ill, and most do. Their growth is so rapid that the acid-alkaline balance of their bodies is easily disturbed, becoming overacid and creating the basis for infection.

Breast-Feeding

The infant's diet is of prime importance, followed closely by his psychic environment. Does mother kiss the knee when it gets bumped? Is the child supported, loved, accepted, appreciated? These acts of love affect children at the level of the thymus or heart center and actually help their immune system. The immune system, however, receives its biggest boost from the time-honored custom of breast-feeding. As family doctors, Gladys and I have always urged mothers to breast-feed their children, and in our own family all six children were breast-fed at least for a while. Our clinical experience has been that breast-fed babies were not as sickly as those who were bottle-fed—neither during the first few months of their lives nor later, after the breast and the bottle were discarded. Recently there has been research evidence from Columbia University as well as from some Swedish pediatricians (*Medical Tribune*, October 12, 1977) that this clinical observation is further supported in the laboratory.

The mammary gland, according to Dr. Jane Pitt, is an immunologic organ, and it appears that there are almost as many antibody-containing lymphocytes or lymph cells in human milk as in the peripheral bloodstream. The breast-fed infant, it seems, is continuously furnished with the capacity to resist whatever pathogens may come his way. Why is this? New evidence from Sweden reveals that nursing mothers are colonized with the very microorganisms that their babies meet up with in this postbirth or neonatal period. Dr. Pitt says this is a change from prior thinking, when it had been thought that babies were colonized by their mothers. Apparently, immunization may take place directly in the breast tissue, or via the alimentary canal (gut) itself. Dr. Pitt and her colleagues are just beginning to recognize the phenomenon of "homing," whereby compartments of the immune system—such as the gut and the breast—may be intercommunicating with each other.

A study done by Dr. Alan Cunningham of some 253 infants in 1974, in Cooperstown, New York, showed that the incidence of all illnesses proved to be two or three times higher among bottle-fed than breast-fed infants. This held true for both high- and low-income families. Admissions to the hospital were eight to nine times more frequent among the bottle-fed babies. Further, among bottle-fed babies there was twice as much otitis media, fifteen times as much lower respiratory illness, and two and a half times as much gastrointestinal sickness.

Thus, we see how the urging of many family physicians for the new mother to breast-feed her baby has gained research support. It makes sense, since breasts were formed for this purpose, and the mother's milk obviously has purpose and value for the infant.

Whether your baby has been breast-fed or not, common infections and problems are bound to arise. When one of these common problems begins, that is the best time to take steps to cure the early infection.

Castor Oil Therapy

We have found that castor oil applications and Glycothymoline packs or drops are among the most widely used and probably the most effective therapies. We have used castor oil packs regularly for diarrhea and colic and we have used castor oil drops in children's ears. We have used castor oil packs for sore throats, appendicitis in early stages, and hyperkinesis (the hyperactive child). Finally, we have applied castor oil locally to many parts of the body for bruises, scrapes, and puncture wounds.

One seventeen-year-old patient who had cut his right ankle on a piece of glass had it repaired at the emergency room of Scottsdale Baptist Hospital. There was such extreme sensitivity and pain that he had to use crutches to get around. When I saw him three days later, his entire ankle hurt and the wound was painful to the touch. It was not infected, but I felt that the nerve supply to that area had been injured and possibly a ligamentous laceration had produced such extreme symptoms. In any event, he was instructed how to use castor oil packs over the wound. Two days later he felt markedly better and was able to go without crutches. After seven days, sutures were removed, and our seventeen-year-old was back playing football six days later. Instead of sensitivity around the wound area, there was now just a bit of numbness, and our patient was told to continue massaging the area with the oil until the numbness was gone.

Appendicitis remains a difficult problem both to diagnose and to treat in the practice of medicine. Several years ago, an eleven-year-old patient developed classical signs of an inflamed appendix. Castor oil packs overnight maintained a state of semi-status quo. His white blood cell count was only 5,300 with 70% polys; and urine showed a few white cells and a trace of albumen. Sixteen hours after onset, acupuncture was accomplished just below stomach point #36, with relief of much of the tenderness. There was no vomiting, but there was a low-grade fever of 99.8°. Diet consisted of only small amounts of clear liquids. Surgical consultation at twenty-four hours postonset produced strong recommendations that surgery be done. However, the parents declined, feeling that there was sufficient reason to expect recovery. Another acupuncture was done at thirty hours after onset. After another night with continued packs, all symptoms and abnormal findings were gone by the next morning. The patient resumed his activities with no subsequent problem, and a follow-up blood count was normal.

This case clearly supports my observations written in *Edgar Cayce and the Palma Christi*, where twelve of thirteen cases clinically diagnosed as appendicitis were cleared using only castor oil packs, with ice chips and sips of fluid as the only diet. Castor oil packs in a routine of three times a week were suggested for a four-month follow-up to aid in preventing any further attacks.

A young couple wrote me when their one-year-old boy could not find relief for five to six months of chronic, persistent diarrhea. Having known them for several years, I wrote to them about the castor oil packs, and the possibility of using Glycothymoline packs also. They later wrote me that he was now twenty-two months and had no problems with his general intestinal (G.I.) tract. It had cleared up completely just from using castor oil packs.

Otitis media or inflammation of the ear in a one-year-old child is sometimes difficult to combat. Children, as a rule, are more subject to such infectious diseases than are their adult counterparts. A registered nurse on the East Coast wrote to me that her baby had developed ear trouble at the age of nine months. Her pediatrician had given her antibiotics and a decongestant. One month's treatment found the infant with fluid behind the left tympanum and a residual inflammation. A change of decongestants for another month left the other ear even more inflamed, bringing about still another change of decongestant plus a promise of a visit to an otologist if the ears had not cleared in another three weeks, with drainage tubes likely to be inserted at that time. It was at this point that our correspondence started. Drawing on my experience in the field of healing and with the Cayce material, I wrote as follows:

> Briefly, I think these things might be helpful as far as your baby is concerned. I would try to get her on a very alkaline diet. This is a bit difficult for a one-year-old baby but I think it would be important. Then castor oil drops in the ears at bedtime and early in the morning; Glycothymoline packs to the neck for half an hour or so once a day with packs going around including the cervical glands. She should have lots of vitamin C—I think you can get this in liquid form now and high dosages of this would be helpful.

> Massages to the upper back for fifteen to twenty minutes each day gently would be a good thing and castor oil packs to the abdomen. This should also be done once a day for about an hour and I would use the heating pad.

> Don't forget that the laying on of hands by those who love the child is part of the whole process of healing, and if you're involved in the healing profession as you are, you should certainly be doing this sort of thing. The thing I would suggest is to have your daughter lie on your lap as she goes to sleep, in taking her afternoon nap or whatever, and hold your hands on her head behind the ears encompassing the ears. She might not like to have ears covered with your hands but if she doesn't mind that would be good. Then just let yourself be a channel of healing and let the energy flow through your body and onto the ears themselves.

> Doing these things over a period of time would be very helpful I'm sure.

It was two months before I heard what had happened. The mother answered for the daughter at that point and expressed the daughter's approval of the program of therapy. Her letter:

The baby is fine now; her ears have cleared up completely. Just before I received your letter, I had started giving her increased doses of vitamin C, rubbing some castor oil over her abdominal area at night, and saturating the front of her diaper with castor oil as well. However, I did not use heat. I also gave her a little Glycothymoline occasionally by mouth because I felt she had a tendency to be acid. As soon as I received your letter I began adding your suggestions to these treatments. When I took her back to the doctor a few days later, he was surprised to find that her ears had cleared up completely. Her improvement was especially disconcerting to him since she had refused his prescribed medicine since her last visit to his office. Thank you for your time and information. —Our love and blessings . . .

It was nearly twelve years ago that Gladys used castor oil packs on a hyperactive child for the first time, and that was not because of the hyperkinesis, but because five-year-old Jimmy complained to his mother that he had a sore tummy. When examined in our office, the boy did not show any signs of appendicitis or of any significant problem, but was given the packs because they usually dispense stomach discomfort in children. During his time in the examining room, Jimmy was total destruction. He had everything in an uproar, much like many hyperactive children. However, by the time of his second visit, after a month of taking the castor oil packs on his tummy, Jimmy was a changed boy. He acted like a normal child, not tearing pages out of magazines, not opening and closing doors and drawers, etc.

From that time on, we came to use these castor oil packs on a number of children with disturbances of the nervous system. The packs seemed always to have a quieting, healing effect. In the mid-1970s,

Dr. Ernie Pecci was involved in some related research treating sixteen children who exhibited "minimal brain dysfunction." The children were treated at the Contra Costa County daycare centers in Oakland, California, where Ernie is medical director. Half of them were given a regimen of castor oil packs over the abdomen, a special diet, and supplementation with vitamins E and C, plus a multiple vitamin, and the other half remained untreated over the five-week test period. The children in both groups were tested in several ways, both before and after the test period. Parents were involved in the evaluation together with teachers and psychologists. No world-shaking events were uncovered in that short period of time, but some six of the eight children given the treatment package were improved. The results reported were interesting: sleeping patterns were improved; weight gain was noted in some; a reduction in hyperactivity was common; skin color or complexion improved; memory was better; they were calmer; talks were more related; and one noted that his vision somehow "appears improved."

Retardation

After borrowing the Circulating File on Mongolism: Children, Abnormal, an A.R.E. member reported on what she had done with it. Apparently, she could not find a doctor who would work with her on care of her newborn infant, who had this problem. So she proceeded to do something herself. It reminds me of what Cayce said so often: it is better to do anything, even if it is wrong, than to do nothing at all. Well, this woman did something, but it was not wrong for the child. Here is her story:

> You asked how this file helped—our baby is a Downs Syndrome and for the first six months of his life we massaged him nightly with equal parts of olive, peanut, and castor oils. We are now taking him twice weekly to an A.R.E. cooperating chiropractor for the Cayce recommended adjustments. We are much encouraged—the baby is alert,

responsive—his appetite and eliminations have improved—he's stronger physically and his gift to us on his first birthday, 8/29/75; was to clap hands when we asked him to do "patty cake." We are grateful to Him for His "amazing grace."

A child who has been diagnosed as having cerebral atrophy and an organic brain syndrome does not have a bright outlook. However, when parents work with such a child consistently, patiently, and persistently, things do happen.

From the multitude of readings Cayce gave about children who were brain-injured or retarded, there was always the admonition that those who were given care over these children be loving and prayerful as they sought to bring them back to a normal condition; and they were always instructed to be patient, persistent, and consistent in all that they did for them.

Child Care

Baby care certainly becomes a loving care over a lifetime in some instances; however, most problems are not that large, and fortunately they can be solved through the judicious use of common sense and some simple suggestions. A Circulating File on Baby Care is available through the A.R.E. membership department, and many members have used suggestions found there in care of their own children. Such an example of research at the grassroots level comes from Cleveland:

Becoming A.R.E. members just recently, this is the first time my husband and I have really worked with the physical readings. . . . Well, I'm very happy to announce that by following a reading from the Baby Care series (General), I used Carbolated Vaseline for our infant daughter's skin irritation (facial). She breaks out on the face, I feel, from just the irritation of milk she has spit up which gets on the face. This Vaseline cleared her up within twenty-four hours and I now use it as a preventive measure to protect her skin. I suggested this to my sister-in-law who used the Vaseline, also, for a *severe* case of diaper rash. Her daughter was helped too. (My daughter is three months old.) I had used various types of baby creams before the Carbolated Vaseline and *none* of them helped.

Warts present a problem to most mothers as their children grow up. And the problem exists for the doctor, too, because they are often difficult to cure. One such patient several years ago failed to respond to castor oil applied time after time. The father then took things into his own hands, rubbed a potato slice on the warts (like his own mother did when he was a child) and buried the potato out in the yard, when no one else was watching. The warts immediately started going away, and within a two-week period they had disappeared!

I remember reading in the *British Medical Journal* the method one doctor reported—his way of removing warts from the gullible four-, five-, or six-year-old was to pay them sixpence for each wart. It worked. But the price has probably gone up by now.

Pinworms in the child have been indicated as causative of irritability, hyperactivity, inattention in school, loss of appetite, and lack of sleep, resulting in learning difficulties. It has been said that a tenth of the population of our country suffers from infection with this intestinal parasite. There have been many suggestions offered to prevent reinfection and passage of the eggs to other individuals, all of these ideas centering around cleanliness. Cleanliness is next to Godliness, if we believe our biblical instructions, but there are ideas found in the Cayce readings that rarely deal with cleanliness. If you obtain the Circulating File on Worms: Pinworms, reading 2015–10 will supply you with some fascinating information. This three-year-old girl had a number of problems, but apparently the intestinal pinworms were causing her most of her difficulty at the time the reading was given. The three questions tell an interesting story:

Q-3: Are the bones of her feet normal? Does she have flat feet or fallen arches, that her shoes won't stay on, or she won't allow them to stay on?

A-3: As we find, these are normal in the present. This is the natural tendency of the body. We will find that with the removal of these tendencies in the intestines, that tendency for the body to turn its toes down, or in, will be eliminated.

Q-4: How did the trouble of pinworms originate, or what caused it?

A-4: Milk! You see, in every individual there is within the intestinal tract that matter which produces a form of intestinal worm. This is in everyone. But with a particular diet where the milk has any bacillus, it will gradually cause these to increase, and they often-times develop or multiply rapidly; and then they may disappear, IF there is taken raw, green food.

Q-5: Would you change the kind of milk she drinks?

A-5: It isn't so much the change in the kind of milk that is needed. Either add the raw, green foods as indicated, or give those properties as would eliminate the sources of same. But it is better, if it is practical, to induce the body to eat lettuce and celery and carrots—even a small amount. One leaf of lettuce will destroy a thousand worms.

Cayce upsets all conventional medical thought concerned with etiology of this common condition—the idea that the body can create and in fact *does* create pinworms capable of producing eggs and reproducing themselves is worthy of the concept that man is a creative individual, indeed. Perhaps worthy of a healthy skepticism is the concept in the third answer Cayce gave for this little girl—that worms in the intestinal tract would make her turn her toes in or down and that administration of lettuce will keep her shoes on her feet. Strange, this human body—is it not?

In other readings for pinworms, Cayce suggested cabbage as well as lettuce and raw vegetables like carrots and celery plus raw fruit. Perhaps we in the United States do not give our children enough of those raw foods? The following story came to me from a correspondent in Birmingham who had a problem with pinworms in her family several years ago:

> I used to spend a good deal of money on medications. The whole family had to be treated if one person had the worms—boiled clothing and sleepless nights.
>
> Somewhere I read in the Cayce readings about eating raw cabbage and cut out milk for a little while, and if we needed help from then on, I went for the cabbage treatment right away and the persons involved were free of worms right away. We had three girls at the age when the oldest started school. That is when we started our pinworm problem, but can guarantee that the cabbage helped, with no milk but juices instead for a few days.

Injuries cause a great deal of difficulty among children. When a child is involved in an accident, sometimes serious injuries such as cerebral concussion can come about. In understanding this kind of injury, it is best to look at it as a continuous process in the living organism instead of as a single event in time. A physical trauma always brings on the condition we might diagnose as a concussion, but the cells within the body are constantly changing, and the effect of the injury is either increasing the total body discomfort and pathological state of the nervous system, or the body as a whole is cleaning up the debris, in effect, and making the body near whole again.

Some years ago, I hospitalized a twelve-year-old girl who had been struck by an automobile while she was riding her bike. She was unconscious for five or ten minutes but recovered enough to talk coherently, and we discovered no obvious fractures.

Her X-rays in the hospital revealed a hairline skull fracture, however, and she was kept very quiet. As the evening wore on, she became more and more lethargic, lapsing into a coma gradually. I had started her on injections of an enzyme preparation that was in common use at that time, for I felt that if there was swelling of the tissues or any minimal bleeding into the tissue of the brain, this would aid the body in the healing process. We also had some study groups alerted, so they were praying for her. Between ten and eleven-thirty that night, our patient was comatose, and we were ready to call in neurosurgeons, when she began to stir once again. Gradually she regained consciousness, becoming more and more alert, until by morning she was as frisky as she had been before she was struck by the car.

I can just imagine the variety of physiological activities that went on inside her body during those few critical hours. We still do not know whether it was the enzymes or the prayers that turned the tide, or whether it was a spontaneous thing influenced by neither of the two. The result, however, was gratifying.

We recently received a letter from a friend of ours in California. Her six-year-old son took a nasty spill on his bike. Her written story follows:

He had a "goose egg" partially over his right temple and surrounding area. I checked his eyes, and they seemed to focus all right. I asked him if he wanted to go to church or stay home. He opted to go to church . . . but instead of going to his class, he stayed with me, head in my lap. When we got home he complained of not feeling well, and vomited. In talking to him, I discovered he couldn't remember what had happened from the time he fell off his bike till sometime on the way to church. I was very concerned by this time—felt he must have a minor concussion. I put a castor oil pack on the bruise and around his head, and asked him to lie down, and remain comparatively quiet. If I recall correctly, in about an hour and a half, he was asking for something to eat, playing a

game on the bed with his sister—and when I
checked the swelling, it was all gone. I removed
the pack, and he got up. That night I put it back
on until morning. No repercussions that I could
see.

Therapy for children? . . . A mother's concern, a
youth's ability to recuperate, a prayer, and castor oil
. . . And do not underestimate any one of them!

Chapter Twenty Seven
LIFE-THREATENING CONDITIONS

It is probably unwise to call any condition of the
body incurable, for strange things have happened in
the course of human events. For practical purposes,
however, there are conditions that regularly resist
successful therapy and as a result are thought of as
incurable; and many individuals so afflicted are not
cured and their physical bodies do die. Yet, even
when death is near, there is still aid that can be
brought to ease pain and make life more livable
right up to the very end.

Pain in the terminal cancer patient is perhaps the
most feared complication of that disease in the human body. One wonders where pain actually has its
origin—for pain is perhaps the most difficult symp-
tom to pin down and the least understood. In my
own experience with cancer patients who were too
far advanced with the disease to be helped by any of
the available cancer therapies, I have seen some traditional aids bring much relief from pain during the
final days.

In 1975, a sixty-two-year-old man developed a cancer of the brain. By the time he came under medical
observation, it was quite advanced; then a second
malignancy was discovered in the wall of the bladder,
and the only help available was chemotherapy. When
the family consulted us, the patient was terminal, in

bed, experiencing pain, and obviously did not have much time left. He was advised to use castor oil packs on the abdomen, and he remained pain-free until twenty-four hours before he passed away. Then he developed some pain in one flank, and when a castor oil pack was applied locally there, too, he became comfortable once again.

Another instance of the use of these packs came nearly twenty years ago, when I was called upon to care for a woman who had a massive abdominal cancer that was far advanced when I first saw her. She had become unable to care for herself. She refused surgery of any kind and went into a rest home since she had no living relatives. There, she received coffee enemas and abdominal castor oil packs daily for the next forty days until her death. She had no pain at any time.

Another story of the unpleasant, life-threatening complications of cancer came from one of our cooperating physicians. His patient was a thirty-three-year-old woman, two years after a radical mastectomy had been performed. She had been given everything in those two years: surgery, cobalt, radiation, betatron, 5FU, and other chemotherapy. She started losing ground, developing peptic ulcers and elimination problems. Finally she developed abdominal distension and became disoriented and out of touch with reality. After hospitalization, she was started on castor oil packs over the entire abdomen. Her urinary tract started working again, and the distension gradually subsided. She was still impacted, but on the fourth day, she started having some bowel activity. On the fifth day, she had her first regular bowel movement in weeks. Her hallucinations cleared up, her vision clinically improved considerably, and she was able to go home from the hospital.

Castor oil packs certainly will not clear up the malignancy we call cancer, but if it can aid the sensorium like it did in this woman and bring about such a significant improvement of the eliminations, then the packs have done something very worthwhile for an individual who is preparing to enter the other side of life through the birth that we call death.

For, in the concept of the continuity of life that we have explored in this book, death becomes the great healer. When an individual experiences the life events that teach him the lessons he came here to learn, then his soul knows that he is ready to go to the other side. Birth there is death here; so we might look at it as saying that birth on the other side of life becomes the healing of the infirmities that we have found to be part of our life experiences here.

When we treat people who have developed one of this group of problems that we might call incurable—cancer, multiple sclerosis, amyotrophic lateral sclerosis, narcolepsy, epilepsy, and many others—it is important that we clarify exactly what we are attempting to do. We must make a choice. Will we:

(1) Treat the disease? Or (2) Treat that person, recognizing that that individual is body, mind, and spirit, and is an adventurer on Earth?

We may choose to treat just the disease or both, if we have the training, expertise, and license; but to treat the *whole* person is another thing. It may involve simply being kind. I remember one of the statements that Cayce made to an individual who was caring for her son who was mentally ill: "The greatest thought that can come to the mind of man is—'Someone cares.' " (3365–1) Treating another person may mean praying for him, physically aiding him in one way or another. Or it may mean using an age-old aid to the physiology of the body that helps his own body to gain back at least partially toward normal.

Applying a castor oil pack, altering a diet, instituting an exercise program, praying for a person, or giving him an enema does not require a license to practice medicine. However, for those who are doctors, Felix Marti-Ibanez had something to say about caring for those who might tend to be hopeless in their attitudes. He was talking to new graduates in medicine:

Your duty to your patients will be to act toward them as you would wish them to act toward you: with kindness, with courtesy, with honesty. You

must learn when and how to withhold the truth
from your patients if by not telling them all the
facts of the case you can relieve or console them,
for you can cure them sometimes, you can give
them relief often; but hope you can give them
always. Remember that a laboratory report is not
an irrevocable sentence; behind all such reports
and data, there is a human being in pain and
anguish, to whom you must offer something more
than an antibiotic, an injection, or a surgical aid;
you must, with your attitude, your words, and
your actions, inspire confidence and faith and
give understanding and consolation.

In his readings for those who were ill and suffering from a multitude of conditions, Edgar Cayce
frequently saw that an individual had only a short
period of time to live. Sometimes he said that nothing could be done; but then he invariably went on to
tell those caring for the person what they could do to
aid the patient in making the transition. He always
placed before people the nature of their being—that
they were eternal creatures and that all parts of life,
the good and the bad, the health and the sickness,
were part of that soul's adventure.

Where help could be given, the help—even in the
"incurable" diseases—was aimed toward upgrading the
physiology of the body. Cayce did recommend surgery
at times, and he did suggest X-ray therapy, penicillin,
and other items to meet the "needs of the condition"
as he saw it. Most of the treatments he suggested,
however, were of the type that would make the body
function better and thus overcome its imbalances
and its incoordinations and restore itself to normal.

Multiple Sclerosis

Multiple sclerosis (M.S.) is one of those illnesses
where efforts are made to aid the glands of the body
toward better functioning and to regenerate tissue
that, in the nervous system, is deficient. Multiple
sclerosis is a disease of remissions and aggravations.
It comes and goes, in a sense, leaving the patient

debilitated now and restored back near to normal the next time one measures his condition. It is felt that it is the lack of electrical coherence caused by the myelin sheaths on the nerves that causes such vacillation. These sheaths are affected by the disease and apparently get better, then become worse again. It is important to the proper transmission of impulses that the myelin sheaths are intact.

Suggestions from the Cayce material included diet, wet-cell-battery treatments, and massages. The wet cell battery uses a weak electrical current, and the story that comes from the Cayce readings is that electricity, no matter what its source, is working with life forces, especially if it is the "low" form of electrical energy. Cayce suggested, in the case of one who was told to use the wet cell, that there are elements in the earth from which and to which every atom of the body responds. This man, only thirty-two years old, was given the following suggestion:

> We would use the low Wet Cell Appliance, as this produces that vibration nearer to life energy itself in human experience. For, all life is electrical energy. That produced as life force is from the combinations of the principal elements in the Wet Cell Appliance, preparing in the manner as has been indicated, in the right proportions for the regular charge.

3491–1

Many individuals with M.S. arrive at the Clinic, and many of them see Dr. Ray Bjork at least once while they are here. Often, Ray will bring Mabel, his wife, into the consultation room with him, for they have worked together on these problems for twenty years or more, ever since Ray was striken with M.S. and had to quit active medical practice. He and Mabel applied the concepts and therapies found in the Cayce readings on his own body, and he improved enough that he could come back to active work in the Clinic. He still sees patients in consultation occasionally, even though he is retired and in his mid-seventies.

An extract from a letter written recently by the wife of one of Ray's patients is most revealing:

> As I said on the phone, Bruce has had no M.S. attacks in a year and a half (he had been having them once to twice yearly) and has learned to listen to what his body is telling him. When he's tired he knows it's time to quit and not press on. He follows a low-fat diet (Swank diet) and recently learned that his cholesterol reading is 130—not bad!
>
> Bruce found his introduction to the techniques of meditation (while in Phoenix) particularly valuable. He has learned to combine his time with the wet cell with meditation that has markedly changed his life in many ways. Your wonderful letter makes us realize that you have a deep faith in God's healing power, as we do.

Narcolepsy

Narcolepsy is uncommon but not rare in the experience of the physician. It can be caused by structural lesions affecting the nervous system and causing excessive sleepiness. These are the so-called secondary types of narcolepsy. The "primary" syndrome is the usual case, and its cause in the textbooks of medicine is unknown. It ranges from somewhat embarrassing episodes of drowsiness during lectures or after-dinner conversations to severe sleepiness in which subjects spend nearly the entire day drifting in and out of sleep. When a pattern has been established early in life, it often continues without letup throughout the person's normal life, unless treated with stimulants to prevent sleep. This therapy is not always successful, and it has its own set of side-effects.

In the Cayce material, at least one type of narcolepsy seemed to have its origin in a disturbance of a portion of the glandular system. The following extract is from a reading given to a thirty-year-old woman.

Q-5: Sleepiness?

A-5: This comes from the fagging of the nerves and muscular forces; and we will find there will be corrections in these directions as the general health is improved, and as this slowing of circulation to the superficial portion of the body is corrected.

Q-6: Is the recent appearance of the sleepy feeling from the same cause as that when I was 17, when I slept practically one whole summer?

A-6: Partially; though then it was more acute than it has reached in the present. Glandular disturbance and slowing of superficial circulation, with the lack of carrying energies to the locomotories of the body.

Q-7: Is this akin to sleeping sickness?

A-7: Yes, it might be said to be a double-first cousin.

2769–1

Nearly six months ago, a forty-year-old woman was examined at the A.R.E. Clinic for what had been diagnosed as narcolepsy of four years' duration. She found that she experienced cataleptic seizures (a trancelike condition of the body, with rigidity of the muscles) when she laughed vigorously. This is one of the diagnostic findings, and had been characteristic of her history for three years before she was seen here. She had taken a variety of stimulants that kept her going but did not really keep her awake. She has had several acupuncture treatments, but to no avail.

Her treatment was designed around the concept that this disease is in reality caused by a glandular imbalance, as Cayce suggested. It is interesting that the catalepsy comes about when the patient laughs— that is emotion, isn't it? The patient was started on Atomidine in increasing dosage. Over the next month she upped her dosage to ten drops daily for five days out of the week. This was supported by the use of castor oil packs, exercises in walking, and some yoga that she was interested in. Her catalepsy stopped immediately. She rapidly developed a normal energy pattern and reported four months after starting the treatment that she had not felt as good and full of energy since her children were small (some twelve to fifteen years previously), and she was then able to work normally without tiring. The Cayce readings imply that Atomidine is valuable in treating a glandular deficiency.

Epilepsy

Epilepsy is another illness that should be included in this chapter, for it is rare that one can be completely cured of this disease by traditional methods. Over the centuries, epilepsy has been associated with genius—that is, up until the last five or six decades, when drugs came into common use. Less and less has it been possible for these unnumbered, unrecognized budding geniuses to reach their potential, due to the sedative and toxic effects imposed on them by the use of drugs such as phenobarbital and diphenylhydantoin. Because of the fear of convulsions, and because these drugs lessen the number and severity of convulsions, patients have been almost universally accorded their use.

In our continuing study of epilepsy and the use of a therapy approach suggested from the Cayce material, we have found that a new, bright, creative individual arises out of the obscurity of the drugged state. When patients suffering from convulsive disorders are started on castor oil packs, a good low-carbohydrate diet, massages, and the proper use of attitudes and supportive emotional care, the old concept that many geniuses also had epilepsy becomes more evident. The drugs in reality do suppress mental functioning. When one considers the rationale behind the use of castor oil packs over the abdomen as it is expressed in the Cayce readings, one has the opportunity to make that difficult choice between a regenerative approach to the problem or the use of drugs.

One of our cooperating doctors worked with a nine-year-old girl who had been diagnosed as epileptic some four years earlier. Since then, she had been on Dilantin, and her mother described her as nervous, crying often, and tending toward panic in tense situations. She had complained almost constantly about stomachaches and a fuzziness in her right foot. She was then subjected to a changed therapy program.

For two months, she was given regular castor oil packs, massages, manipulations, and a fairly strict dietary regimen. Her teacher volunteered the information that she was "a changed person from the beginning of the year." She was considerably more relaxed; she had a happy attitude; she had no more nightmares, which had once plagued her; and her color was better. She no longer had the stomachaches or the fuzziness in the foot that had bothered her. In spite of the fact that she was still on Dilantin, her changes in awareness, general health, and symptomatology spoke highly of what had been done for this young lady in just a period of two months. The parents are continuing with the treatments, and hopefully they will do so for a long enough period of time so that a full healing can come about.

Cancer

The literature on cancer would undoubtedly fill thousands of bookshelves. Here on these few pages is some information that will simply make you think, and be helpful if you are faced with caring for someone with cancer. There is something about the nature of cancer that needs to be put into context with regard to the nature of the human being. Out of some ideas that stimulate or shock a bit may come a helpful concept of what to do with the cancer patient who has received all that he can or will receive as far as treatment of the cancer itself is concerned.

You may have cancer—and never know it, and even be ill with it! This is the controversial statement coming from a UCLA researcher, Jean deKernion. Speaking to a group of physicians, deKernion pointed out that the natural defenses of the body overcome the malignancy (*Arizona Republic*, March 19, 1978). "Tumors have antigens which are not found in normal cells. This alerts the body's defense system to regard the tumor as a foreign invader and attack it," deKernion said. "The effectiveness of that attack determines whether or not the cancer will be conquered."

Much has been learned over the years about the "defense system" of the body—the thymus is the control tower and the reticuloendothelial system is the home ground where the lymphocytes and the larger mononuclear cells plan war on the invaders. The body is the battlefield. Only usually the cancer cell is not an invader—it is just an undernourished normal cell that goes wild and starts fighting the world around it. There is not enough oxygen, perhaps, or not enough of something vital, to keep the cell normal. It is then that the defense system goes after the errant cell and usually destroys it. If the defense is unsuccessful, the cancer cell proliferates and spreads its influence and its territory, finally destroying the body if not stopped.

What is deKernion's solution when the defense system fails? BCG, perhaps; cell extracts taken from animals who have cancer; serum from cured cancer patients; spleen and lymph-node extracts taken from sheep after the animals have been injected with human cancer cells. Problems, he said, exist with all of these methods, and the answer has not yet been found.

One source of help that researchers such as deKernion have not investigated is the indwelling capacity of the system itself to respond to thought, to suggestion, to general upgrading of the body health, and to the administrations given by those who are said to be healers. However, it seems we are making ground in this direction. Work such as that done by Carl Simonton in Fort Worth has shown that visualization increases the ability of the body to overcome cancer. Looking at this body of evidence only, without even considering the numerous reported cases of spontaneous remission of cancer by those who have been prayed for or who were fasting, it becomes evident that the possibility exists that one can alter the destiny of the cancer cells simply by altering the state of mind or emotions of the human body.

In the Edgar Cayce material, things are taken a step further, beyond the mind-emotion-body relationship, to include the nature of the human being in the first place—his spiritual state. One of the readings that I have valued for a long time speaks to this state of being for each of us, relating us to the Creative Forces and indicating that there is a value in living that must be sought, or else we create situations that become destructive to us, which we call illness. Cayce's viewpoint that there are many lives that we all experience lends an overview to this perspective that makes it a bit more understandable.

Q-5: Will I ever get well?

A-5: Will tomorrow ever come? This depends upon purposes, aims, desires, hopes and fears! Does the body desire to get well? Is God in His heaven? Are the lives and activities of those ye touch helped through the spreading of His work? Do you need to get well? These are all answered in self. He withholds no good thing from those who serve Him. Let ALL remember that, believe it, know it! For it IS the truth! Each illness, each disturbance is sin at thy door!

                                                   2526–5

We all are basically concerned with this life; and once we have agreed that there is purpose in living, and take steps to implement the inferences of that belief, we want to overcome the problem that is facing us. I have always been impressed by the idea that a good offense is the best defense. Not everyone subscribes to it, but if you want to see what the offense amounts to within your own body, you should see the film available through the American Cancer Society called "The Embattled Cell." It is a fascinating time-lapse movie showing the lymphocytes within living tissue in the act of destroying cancer cells. They act intelligently, and, given enough assistance, they could certainly do what they often are unable to do—namely, destroy the cancer within the body before the cancer cells get a real foothold. That would explain how many of us have some of those cancer cells within us right now, and the active, vital lymphocytes are winning the battle and destroying them; and all the while, we are consciously unaware of what is going on.

David Weiss and his coworkers, immunologists at the Hebrew University of Jerusalem in Israel, feel that cancer occurs when the body's immunological system breaks down. Their efforts have been directed toward improving the body's defense system and letting that system destroy the cancer. They have taken white blood cells from animals with cancer, incubating these in a culture with the actual cancer cells. They have then added what they think is the key factor, MER (methyl alcohol extraction residue), which is made from the same bacteria used to make the BCG vaccine, which has the ability to stimulate the immunological system. The white cells are stimulated by this technique in their ability to fight foreign material in the body—their initial responsibility—and they are then returned to the same animal's bloodstream where they selectively go after the cancer cells. They are enormously successful in destroying the animal cancers, according to Weiss. The white blood cells are given, in other words, a chemical education, then are sent out to do their job on the cells that they are now able to overcome. They really recognized them before, for they destroyed part of the cells, but now they are armed. A fascinating concept, is it not?

Dr. Edmund Klein of Buffalo, New York, did some work like this several years ago. He took white blood cells from patients whose skin cancers had been treated successfully with certain drugs applied to the skin. During treatment with these drugs, Dr. Klein claims, their white cells have learned to recognize the cancer cells as foreign tissue and to attack them. When these "educated" cells are then given to other patients who have the same kind of skin cancer, their own white cells quickly pick up the message of how to recognize skin cancer cells, and so become mobilized to destroy them. The teaching process takes only five hours—then the body's lymphocytes have learned how to search out and destroy the cancer cells.

If these reports—and literally hundreds of others— do in fact point up the immune system as the key to the body's defense against cancer and the means by which the body may overcome cancer, then how do we increase the capability and the knowledge of that system? Perhaps castor oil packs can be a significant aid. Visualization, prayer, meditation, laying on of hands, herbs, massage, vitamins, general health-building measures, and certainly diet all play their role.

Gastric cancer is not as common in these days as it used to be. But the causation or the factors associated with the incidence of this type of cancer are dramatically pointed up in a paper by Graham and his coworkers (Graham, Schotz, and Martino, "Alimentary Factors in the Epidemiology of Gastric Cancer," *Cancer*, October 1972). These investigators found, for instance, that those people who had developed gastric cancer more frequently than the controls ate more potatoes, avoided lettuce, ate more irregularly, and used cathartics more frequently. Control patients in this series ate larger numbers of vegetables raw than did cancer patients. Low risk of gastric cancer was associated with ingesting raw lettuce, tomatoes, carrots, cole slaw, and red cabbage, and the risk declined with increases in the number of these vegetables eaten raw.

Perhaps the most outstanding recommendation in the Cayce readings for people who had cancer *of any kind* was to move toward a raw vegetable diet; and when a person had a far-advanced cancer, Cayce often suggested that the diet be "that that a cow or a rabbit would eat." The implication from the readings being that not only are such things as green salads highly important in preventing cancer, but that they are helpful in treatment.

For centuries the chaparral plant, which grows so profusely in the deserts of the southwest, has been, for the Indians native to that area, a healing medium that is surpassed by few herbs. In Virginia Sculley's *A Treasury of American Indian Herbs* (Crown Publishers, Inc.), she tells how the Indians used the chaparral plant or creosote bush as a tonic, a cleanser for the kidneys, and, mixed with badger oil, as an ointment for burns. They used it as a tea for colds or for chills, for intestinal trouble, rheumatism, snakebite, tetanus, and sores and bruises. Other sources of information think the chaparral is primarily a stimulant to better liver function. It recently has had an amazing upswing in usage, as modern herbalists have put the leaves together in pressed forms and suggest that it be taken by mouth instead of as a tea. A rather recent story is told of a man with a facial cancer that would have required major surgery in a hospital in Utah. The man declined the surgical treatment and started chaparral tea on the advice of an old Indian friend of his. Some months later, he showed up at the hospital for a reexamination, and his cancer was gone. Chaparral's use against cancer is still being researched. Meanwhile, people with a wide variety of problems are starting to drink chaparral tea once a day. They use it for everything from the common cold and arthritis to cancer.

Linus Pauling and vitamin C are linked closely together in the minds of most Americans since the time, some years ago, when the medical profession argued vehemently against Pauling and his claim that vitamin C was helpful in fighting the common cold. Now comes information from the Linus Pauling Institute of Science and Medicine that should stir even more controversy: vitamin C may help cancer victims. Pauling's institute carried out studies in collaboration with Vale of Leven Hospital in Scotland, publishing the results in the October 1976 issue of the *Proceedings of the National Academy of Sciences*. According to this study, one hundred advanced cancer patients were given ten grams of sodium ascorbate (vitamin C) per day in addition to their normal treatment. The other one thousand patients, suffering from advanced cancer also, received the identical treatment except for the vitamin C. The patients given the vitamin C have lived—on the average—five times as long (after being deemed "terminal") as the matched control patients.

According to a recent report by oncology researchers at the University of Wisconsin and described in *Modern Medicine* (April 15, 1978), vitamin B_6 can prevent recurrences of bladder cancers in some patients. Among 121 subjects suffering recurrence of the disease, who were divided into a test and a placebo group, "the group that received the B_6 definitely had fewer tumors." The test came about after Professor Raymond Brown noted that many bladder cancer victims have B_6 deficiencies. Not all the test group responded with improvement, but there were no toxic side-effects, and the vitamin can be taken orally with ease. The theory about the effect brought about by the B_6 is that it either reduces the carcinogen in the bladder or it strengthens the body's immune system.

Temple Beautiful Program

Many of the chronic, sometimes incurable diseases have not been touched on. So what would or could be done in those instances? It must seem by now pretty obvious that there are certain procedures that anyone can take that will help to restore health to the human being, no matter what is wrong. It may *not* restore complete health, for the individual has creative abilities, and may wish, for some unknown, unconscious reason, to live through the problem he has created within his own body.

How do we, as professionals, deal with problems like this? We usually have patients with life-threatening illnesses come to us already under as much specific therapy as can be obtained. Over the years, we have implemented in our practice one after the other of these supportive concepts we have been discussing. Then, in 1978, we began a group therapy that put together most of these aids in a seventeen-day program that we called the Temple Beautiful Program. It recalls a legendary site of healing in ancient Egypt that Cayce talked about, which was

called the Temple Beautiful. The program was designed to aid each participant in realizing that his
or her body was indeed the real Temple Beautiful, if
steps were taken by them to bring that into reality.

At a recent program, seriously ill (although still
ambulatory) patients numbered seven out of the
eleven enrolled. Four had either preoperative or post-
operative cancer of the breast, one was working with
M.S., one young man had recently developed amyotrophic lateral sclerosis, and another (with familial
kidney disease) was just two weeks away from kidney dialysis. Besides a complete medical workup,
each person was introduced to a nutritional program,
was given massages and colonics, and was taught
autogenic exercises and visualization through biofeedback training and counseling. As a group, they
experienced music and color and dance, and tuned in
to their unconscious minds, using music as the bridge
and art as the medium, and each received a massage
to music by therapists trained in this healing modality.

They dreamed and learned to interpret their dreams,
finding new insights into their attitudes and emotions;
and nearly all experienced real breakthroughs in these
areas. There was the laying on of hands in which
they took part by both giving and receiving; and
prayer and meditation was a regular morning experience. Exercise also became a part of the program,
depending on the state of health of the individual,
and castor oil packs were used. Some are using the
wet cell battery. Past-life experiences were recalled,
helping the participant to look at the past with
understanding, and to the future with promise.

Were these people healed? It is too soon to say,
but I feel that a deep part of each participant underwent a healing process that became part of what we
could call soul growth. Whether this manifests as
physical healing or not will only be told over a much
longer period of time, and it is totally dependent on
that person's will and chosen destiny.

CONCLUSION

At this time, little really remains to be added. A number of illnesses of the body have been touched on from the viewpoint of enhancing the function of the body or what really should be termed its regeneration. Yet, far more of the body difficulties have not even been mentioned, but this was to be expected within the framework of a simple volume, and I make no apologies. Perhaps the stimulation of the mind that comes about when new ideas and new approaches to healing of the body are suggested will prove valuable enough to get you started in better understanding your health and your body.

Many of the therapies that have been identified in these pages may seem outmoded, but I came across something not too long ago that puts medicine of the present day into better perspective and gives us insights that otherwise might pass us by. From the *Today* publication (January–February 1976) of what used to be the Women's Medical College of Pennsylvania, now the Medical College of Pennsylvania, came several items of interest. Paying tribute to the Bicentennial motif, the publication reprinted news items of the day from 1750 and thereabouts, as they pertain to medicine, including the following:

Indians Discover Aspirin
(Also Find Cures for Scurvy and Malaria)

Colonial physicians report learning several important treatments from Indian medicine—the cure for scurvy through the use of the bark of the hemlock-spruce tree and a treatment for malaria from the cinchona in the Peruvian bark with its quinine. The Indian use of a substance known as salicin (aspirin) has also been found effective in reducing the pain of rheumatism.

Along with this recognition of the source of our most common wonder drug, the publication also calls attention (in 1750) to the manner in which colonists were being priced out of the health care market, as medical costs climb and house calls are twenty-five cents per visit. It was at this juncture also (1750) that men broke the taboo against their attendance at childbirth, and the male finally entered the field of obstetrics. "Sometimes gowned in female clothing for the sake of modesty, the male midwives are reported to have greater knowledge and to learn safer techniques—resulting in their growing popularity throughout the colonies."

It's safe to say that in our western civilization much still remains to be discovered and utilized— and perhaps then studied in depth—that pertains to healing of the body. The fact that castor oil was described in the Ebers papyrus and was used as a pack on the abdomen in Europe probably for hundreds of years, and that acupuncture has been used for thousands of years in the Far East, provide us with evidence that the general acceptance or lack of acceptance of a healing modality in our country does not necessarily parallel either its history or its validity.

The Edgar Cayce prescriptions, however, accepted or not by those who make it their business to approve or disapprove, point out a way of life that is truly holistic, identifying man as an eternal creature living here on the planet Earth as body, mind, and spirit. That is why we have called healing an adventure in consciousness, since the process of restoring health is an activity the soul finds itself deeply involved in—and from it, soul growth comes about.

The picture of healing, health, regeneration, longevity, and the human body must all be looked at from a new perspective, if the Cayce material has validity . . . and it does seem to have validity, for when it is used as he suggested it be used, results are forthcoming!

The body can no longer be viewed as a biochemical laboratory, functioning with no particular direction and subject to infirmities from outside. The new picture is one that shows the body to be one with the mind and the spiritual essence—the eternal being—and shows the functioning of the body to be directed by life itself, in the form of electrical, electromagnetic, vibrational energies. The atom itself, the cells of the body, the organs, and the tissues all have consciousness and the possibility to be wholly normal.

There is the reality that each human being may restore his body to a full state of normal, vibrant health. However, there is the caution that such health may come about only in the context of a spiritual origin, a spiritual destiny, and the goals and purposes that must accompany such a state of being. Changes in consciousness, direction, and activity of the body-mind itself are required. For the New Age is saying that we each have a responsibility for our own being, and we really have created what we currently find ourselves doing and being; and that means, among all the rest of the possibilities, our illnesses and our ailments.

How should you use this book for healing in your adventure in consciousness? First, follow these five rules of health in your own life and follow them day by day with persistence, consistency, and patience:

1. Obtain adequate rest for your needs; record and study your dreams.
2. Set up a basic, balanced nutritional program for yourself, and then follow it!
3. Exercise regularly—a little or a lot, but be consistent. And remember that the best exercise is walking.
4. Pray and meditate regularly.
5. Practice the art of using constructive thought, word, and action moment by moment—and continue the process of identifying the difference between that which is constructive and that which is destructive.

Next, review chapter 15, "Putting It All Together." Then, in conjunction with chapter 16, take an inventory of yourself and where you are in consciousness and in body. Finally, do as Mr. Cayce often suggested: begin where you are, use what you have in hand, but start, begin! And then you will be on your way to your own personal adventure in consciousness. Good luck and God bless you.

A WORD ABOUT THE A.R.E. CLINIC

The A.R.E. Clinic of Phoenix, Arizona, is a nonprofit organization dedicated to holistic healing—physical, mental, and spiritual—of the individual. This approach incorporates the best of traditional medicine, New Age healing, and concepts from the Edgar Cayce readings in the fields of patient care, research, and education.

The A.R.E. Clinic was founded in 1970 and grew out of the work of two physicians, Drs. William and Gladys McGarey, and their commitment to research and apply the concepts of health care found in the Edgar Cayce readings. During his lifetime, Cayce gave over fourteen thousand readings that were recorded and transcribed; over nine thousand of these dealt with health, physiology, and healing. Cayce's statement that "spirit is the life-force, mind is the builder, and the physical is the result," accurately describes the Clinic's philosophy of health care.

The name A.R.E. is used through a covenant agreement with the A.R.E.—Association for Research and Enlightenment in Virginia Beach, Virginia—to carry out this work. (The A.R.E. is a membership organization that encourages study, research, and application of the information found in the readings at all levels.)

Today, the breadth of the services offered by the Clinic has expanded to include biofeedback, acupuncture, massage and hydrotherapy, counseling, music, movement and color therapy, osteopathy, diet, meditation, dream study, laying-on-of-hands healing, and therapies from the Cayce readings. The size of the staff has grown from seven in 1970 to nearly forty individuals—doctors, nurses, medical assistants, family nurse practitioners and physicians' assistants, biofeedback and massage therapists, research, education, and administrative personnel. Also, in 1982, a "Center For Regeneration" was opened in Casa Grande, Arizona, on a tract of land given to the clinic.

In addition to offering the "general practice" type of medical care to patients in the Phoenix area, the Clinic offers a variety of programs designed to meet special needs. At Oak House, the Clinic's beautiful residential facility, patients can live and participate in an intensive eight-day or seventeen-day (Temple Beautiful) experience in healing. They will also be part of a group—a small community—that shares meals, exercises, dreams, and supports one another as they change and grow through the duration of the program. Graduates of these programs have reported that they not only experience a greater sense of health and well-being, but that they gain new insights into themselves that help them really to change their lives.

For those individuals enjoying relatively good health who are interested in increasing their own sense of well-being, a new wellness-oriented program in stress management is currently being developed.

For more information, write to the A.R.E. Clinic, 4018 N. 40th St., Phoenix AZ 85018.

INDEX

265

THE WORK OF EDGAR CAYCE TODAY

The Association for Research and Enlightenment, Inc. (A.R.E.®) is a membership organization founded by Edgar Cayce in 1931.

- 14,256 Cayce readings, the largest body of documented psychic information anywhere in the world, are housed in the A.R.E. Library/ Conference Center in Virginia Beach, Virginia. These readings have been indexed under 10,000 different topics and are open to the public.

- An attractive package of membership benefits is available for modest yearly dues. Benefits include: a journal and newsletter, lessons for home study; a lending library through the mail, which offers collections of the actual readings as well as one of the world's best parapsychological book collections; names of doctors or health care professionals in your area.

- As an organization on the leading edge in exciting new fields, A.R.E. presents a selection of publications and seminars by prominent authorities in the fields covered, exploring such areas as parapsychology, dreams, meditation, world religions, holistic health, reincarnation and life after death, and personal growth.

- The unique path to personal growth outlined in the Cayce readings is developed through a worldwide program of study groups. These informal groups meet weekly in private homes.

- A.R.E. maintains a visitors' center where a bookstore, exhibits, classes, a movie, and audio-visual presentations introduce inquirers to concepts from the Cayce readings.

- A.R.E. conducts research into the helpfulness of both the medical and nonmedical readings, often giving members the opportunity to participate in the studies.

For more information and a color brochure, write or phone:

A.R.E., Dept. C., P.O. Box 595
Virginia Beach, VA 23451, (804) 428-3588

ABOUT THE AUTHOR

WILLIAM A. MCGAREY, M.D., received his medical degree from the University of Cincinnati College of Medicine. Since 1964, Dr. McGarey has been Director of Medical Research of The Edgar Cayce Foundation; and since 1970, when The A.R.E. Clinic was formed, has served as its Director and President. In these capacities he has been instrumental in activating research and clinical programs designed to evaluate and utilize concepts in the Cayce readings as they pertain to physiology and therapy. Dr. McGarey is author of *Edgar Cayce and The Palma Christi; Acupuncture and Body Energies;* and coauthor of *Edgar Cayce on Healing;* and coauthor with his wife Gladys, of a book on home and marriage entitled *There Will Your Heart Be Also.* Dr. McGarey is a founding member of The American Holistic Medical Association.